Strength Training Nutrition 101

Build Muscle And Burn Fat Easily…
A Healthy Way Of Eating You Can Actually Maintain

By

Marc McLean
www.weighttrainingistheway.com

Table of Contents

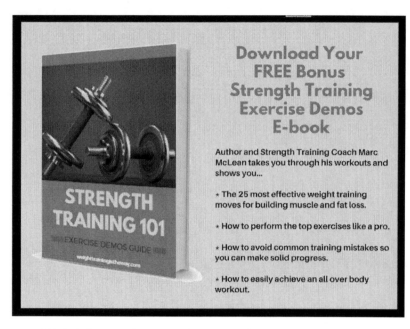

Visit The Website Below To Access Your Copy
www.weighttrainingistheway.com

Introduction

I love food.

I really love it. I know you do too. The health and fitness industry doesn't seem to love it quite so much.

We're bombarded with advice on what we should be eating, how much we should be eating...and what we should be avoiding like an STI.

There are so many diets out there we can't keep up...Paleo, vegan, raw food, SIRT, Atkins, vegetarian, alkaline....I'll leave it there. We could be here a while otherwise. Every diet has its die-hard followers who insist their way is the only way. Not only does this do your head in, it also leaves you confused.

Maybe I shouldn't eat meat? Maybe carbs are the devil? Maybe I should be eating a garden full of greens for breakfast?

This book wasn't written to preach to you about any particular diet. In fact, I hate the word 'diet', I simply prefer a healthier way of eating. Diets are no fun – and most of them don't last.

With the title *Strength Training Nutrition 101*, I reckon you've figured this book is aimed at people who are fond of picking up a dumbbell or two. But I also want to make clear that I won't be regurgitating the usual "you MUST eat six small healthy meals per day" nonsense.

That's what we've heard from 95% of people in the health and fitness industry over the past decade and longer. I've read the same approach in several high profile fitness books and still see it in health magazines, as if it's the only proven way to develop muscle and keep your metabolism at a healthy level to stay lean too.

I tried that approach – eating/grazing every 2-3 hours - for way too many years. Guess what? It left me bloated, miserable and I felt like crap.

Then there's the chicken and broccoli brigade. You see it everywhere on Instagram, people cooking a week's worth of chicken and broccoli, placing it all neatly in 7 containers, and then uploading pictures of said 'prepped' cuisine.

Forget eating the same old, boring, dry, tasteless chicken and soggy greens every day. Think I'd rather become one of those housebound 56 stone men you sometimes see on TV than live like that.

Here's a better idea: how's about we just eat as clean as possible Monday-Friday, limit sugar and booze, live a little more at the weekend, and actually go back to eating our meals in a more normal way?

We've made the uncomplicated way too complicated when it comes to diet and nutrition, particularly for weightlifters looking to gain muscle and strip fat. Want to transform your body and get in better shape? You don't have to go to crazy extremes.

Yes, protein builds muscle – but we don't really need 200, 300...or 400 grams per day like we read about in some fitness magazines. That's just insane.

Yes, energy drinks can give you a boost before your workout. Most of them also contain double the amount of sugar you should have in one day...with ridiculous amounts of caffeine too.

Yes, some supplements can assist in you hitting your health and fitness goals, but what about building a solid nutritional foundation first by eating plenty of whole foods?

The bottom line is that sticking with good nutrition should not be hard work. It should be easy to follow, manageable, and never actually feel like a 'diet'. Since I took up weight training as a ridiculously frail and pale 16-year-old back in 1998, I've experimented with countless ways of eating for energy, performance, muscle gain, keeping my bodyfat levels low and most importantly optimal health.

I've studied various nutritional courses, read countless books and articles, and used myself as a human guinea pig for nearly two decades in the quest for the best approach for all the goals I mentioned above.

The result? I have a formula for eating that is not only healthy, helps me hit all those health and fitness goals...and is <u>easy to maintain</u>. That's the key – if your diet is too complicated or restrictive then you're going to get pissed off in no time and will probably end up going bananas in the nearest Pizza Hut.

In Strength Training Nutrition 101, I share with you how to simplify the way you eat and my golden rules for clean eating. I also reveal my pre-workout nutritional approach that gives me bags of energy and maximises my effort in every workout.

Confused about what you should be eating and when after your gym sessions? I share advice to help you get the most out of all your hard strength training work.

As for supplements, there's so much out there that you could easily spend a fortune. You could also easily waste that fortune. There's a lot of unnecessary, and potentially dangerous, junk out there. You don't need to blow cash on supplements as a proper, healthy diet will give your body the tools it needs to repair, rebuild and remodel your body.

But there are still a handful of (all natural) healthy supplements that I include in my strength training regimen that are really effective. I share my recommended products with you towards the end of the book - and there's also a supplements guide bonus for you for buying this book.

Now onto the main course.

Chapter 1

Simplifying Nutrition For More Muscle and Less Fat

If you're talking to your local gym instructor, personal trainer, or any bodybuilder/powerlifting pals then there's a fair chance they'll say: "Eat regular smaller meals throughout the day, with plenty of protein, that's the way to build and keep muscle."

See, that's the advice that's been spouted for years. Six smaller meals, some even munch through 7 or 8, going crazy for calories and ridiculous amounts of protein to build muscle mass. In fact, I know one bodybuilder who says he eats TEN smaller meals per day and he basically carries plastic tubs of food everywhere with him.

Surely we're verging on ridiculous when it gets to that stage? That just ain't natural. In fact, it's mental. Don't get me wrong, it does work for building muscle. I'm simply arguing that it's not the only way – and that there are a good few downsides to doing it.

You may have been trying to figure out how you're going to manage to prepare and devour so many meals in a day. You may already have been doing it. Prepping food every night or morning, eating by the clock, counting calories and grams of protein like some sort of macronutrients military exercise.

You can choose to do that each day. Every day. Or you can eat in what I consider a more normal way (3-4 meals per day) and still build a strong, athletic, lean physique. I'll also show how eating this way is highly effective for burning fat, while preserving muscle.

I followed the six smaller meals advice for the best part of a decade. Here's what happened...

- It left me feeling bloated all the time.

- The constant clock watching for scheduling meals was monotonous.

- The endless food prepping made me want to chop my own head off.

- I spent way too much time on the toilet.

- I became a slave to my diet.

It was all way too stressful. But I still did it for those 10 years because I thought that was the only way to build muscle and stay in great shape. Looking back on it now, it was nuts.

I changed my mind around 2011, thanks to two people. Kettlebell and hormone optimisation expert Mike Mahler – and my old flatmate Ryan. My friend Ryan moved in with me after splitting up with his girlfriend and he was also into fitness. He also did some weight training and some mixed martial arts too.

Ryan was in great shape and his abs were always ripped. To the point where I considered evicting him. I figured he must train harder, eat better and get in even more protein than I was. So I watched what he was up to – and was pretty shocked.

- While I was stuffing my face with a high protein breakfast within 30 minutes of waking up, Ryan would regularly skip breakfast.

- While I would be munching constantly to cram in calories and protein, Ryan would go long periods between meals and still maintain muscle.

- While I was so strict with my diet and struggled to see my abs, Ryan would occasionally eat junk food and STILL have that damn six pack.

- While I ate all the time, Ryan ate when he was "hungry".

It didn't make any sense. I was the one being mega strict with my nutrition, timing my meals perfectly, a total slave to my diet, and was pretty miserable with it all. Ryan didn't bother with all of that – and was in better shape than me. I remember asking him: "When do you fit in your extra meals? Do you eat a lot when you're at work?"

He said: "No, I don't want to eat 6 or 7 times per day. I eat when I'm hungry and just make sure the food is as healthy as possible."

Around the same time I came across Mike Mahler, an American kettlebell and hormone optimisation expert. Mike follows a vegan diet, eats three or four times per day, and is built like a machine. He also goes against the standard regular smaller meals theory and backs this up through his extensive research on hormones. (Which we'll talk about shortly).

Mike Mahler and my friend prompted me to dig a bit deeper behind their success in staying strong and lean. I found they had the following in common:

- They would take longer stretches between their meals, maybe 5-6 hours. This optimised their hormones, particularly master hormone leptin and increased their insulin sensitivity. (I'll go into more detail on the importance of this later).

- They both managed to get enough calories in over the course of the day to maintain and build muscle. The bigger portion of these were post workout – the prime time for flooding the body with nutrients it needs to repair and build muscle.

- They didn't stress out about meal frequency.

So yeah, I'm going against the grain (pun fully intended) when it comes to the typical diet for men and women looking to gain lean muscle. First, let's talk about the reasons FOR eating 6,7,8 or more smaller meals per day...and then swiftly debunk them.

Main reason #1

"You need to keep supplying your body with calories and protein throughout the day or you'll lose muscle."

A study carried out by 11 sports nutrition experts shows that meal frequency is actually irrelevant, as long as enough calories and the right macronutrients are consumed over course of the day.

Dr John Berardi is founder of Precision Nutrition, who are world leaders in sports nutrition, and he is one of the most highly respected experts on diet and nutrition. He was part of this study and admitted that he too had initially thought that splitting up your daily food intake was the best approach. Dr Berardi said that early research indicated this would speed up the metabolism, help control the hormones insulin and cortisol, and better manage the appetite.

Following their detailed review in the Journal of the International Society of Sports Nutrition, the 11 experts concluded that as long as we eat the right foods in the right amounts, meal frequency is irrelevant. (Further details of this study and other research mentioned later can be found at the end of this book). You can either eat lots of smaller meals every few hours or you can eat a few big meals with bigger breaks in between. It's up to you.

Also debunking the 'eat frequently to maintain muscle' argument is the emergence of The Warrior Diet. Many thousands of people around the world – including big name athletes – are having huge success in sport and developing strong, ripped physiques by following this diet...which is the complete opposite to the eating six or more meals per day. The Warrior Diet, developed by sports scientist and former Israeli Special Forces member Ori Hofmekler, essentially involves fasting for up to 18 hours per day and then feasting at night.

This radical way of eating has been shown to ramp up fat burning, boost energy – while surprisingly preserving muscle mass. There are countless stories of people getting in the best shape of their lives by fasting, or eating very lightly during the day, and then cramming in most of their calories in the evening. This of course also reduces the need for mind-numbing food prepping and eating constantly throughout the day.

The Warrior Diet is followed by sporting superstars including MMA former world champion Ronda Rousey, DC Maxwell, two time women's Jiu-Jitsu world champion, and Pavel Tsatsouline, who basically introduced kettlebell training to the Western world back in 1998. Pavel says he has "better things to do than graze all day".

Main reason #2

"You can't get enough calories in to maintain and build muscle by eating fewer meals per day."

Calories are important, there's no denying that. If you regularly eat too many you'll pile on the pounds. If you don't eat enough you'll lose weight. We get it. There are a few different factors affecting your calorie requirements, but you can roughly figure out how many calories you need using this simple calculation:

Lose weight: bodyweight in lbs x 12 = total number of calories.

Maintain weight: bodyweight in lbs x 15 = total number of calories.

Gain weight: bodyweight in lbs x 17 = total number of calories.

We'll go into more detail about calorie consumption and your body's protein needs a bit later. But first, we're looking at getting in enough calories in just three or four meals rather than six or more. This is simply done in two ways - eating more at each meal and adjusting your diet to include some higher calorie foods. Increasing your intake of healthy fats is a good option as fat provides 9 calories per gram, while protein and carbs provide 4 calories (energy) per gram.

"But won't eating more fat make me fat?"

Not if you eat the right types is the short answer. 'Good' fats are found in fish, plant foods such as nuts, avocados and olives, eggs and dairy. When pulling together your shopping list at the top have foods like salmon, almonds, free range eggs, tuna, olive oil, coconut oil, coconut milk and butter.

There was a long-standing misconception that saturated fats are bad for you when in fact they play several important roles in the body including the manufacture of hormones, stronger bones, boosting the immune system and improved brain health.

Five Reasons Why 3-4 Meals Per Day Is Ideal

So, we've dealt why eating lots of smaller meals every day is not necessary for building and maintaining muscle. Sure, it works – but it can be stressful, difficult to maintain and leaving you feeling like you're chained to a fad diet. Here are five reasons for eating 3-4 meals per day like, erm, most people do.

#1 Taking longer stretches between meals optimises leptin (the master hormone) and keeps insulin sensitive.

Getting down to how diet affects our body at a core level is by looking at our hormones. Hormones are chemical messengers released into the blood which control the functioning of our brain and body. They are responsible for everything from mood and sex drive to physical performance and body composition.

Leptin is a powerful hormone produced in fat cells, which is in control of all other hormones in the body. Eating fewer meals optimises leptin. Eating often, especially with the wrong kinds of foods and in large amounts, causes leptin resistance. This can lead to problems with weight, particularly around the midsection.

Hormone optimisation expert Mike Mahler says that the best way to get out of leptin resistance is to give your body a break from eating large volumes of food often. For those trying to lose fat, sticking with two to three meals per day, with five to eight hours between meals, will give the body an opportunity to use stored bodyfat at energy. For people with lower bodyfat levels and looking to gain more muscle mass, four meals per day with about four hours between meals is a better option.

#2 **To enjoy your food and avoid unnecessary stressing about diet.**

The average person is only awake 16 hours per day so to manage at least six small meals per day you're gonna have to eat every 2.5 - 3 hours. Every day. Every week. This means always keeping an eye on the time to check when your next 'feed' is. It means disturbing your work to snack in the office, eating breakfast as soon as you can after waking up, munching when you're not even hungry, taking food 'on the go' whenever you're out and about, always thinking about what and when you're eating next...

Don't know about you but I'm stressed even reading all of that! How's about we relax and just enjoy three or four meals – when we're actually hungry - instead?

#3 To avoid constant crazy prepping.

When I used to follow the old six-meals-per-day advice I had an entire cupboard full of Tupperware. About 93 tubs of all shapes and sizes – and with countless lids that never seemed to fit. This was for all the 'prepped' small meals I would usually make at night or sometimes in the morning.

I must've wasted about 157.5 days of my life preparing my 'on the go' food. The tuna pasta that I would eat mid-afternoon in between lunch and dinner, or the protein smoothie I would have between breakfast and lunch to bump up the calories and keep feeding my muscle protein. I feared that if I missed a meal my biceps would somehow shrivel up!

One word - insane. Unless you've got your own personal chef, it's a nightmare to keep up with food prepping.

#4 To ease stress on your digestive system.

The length of time it takes to digest food varies from person to person and it also depends on what type of foods you're eating. In a media interview, Dr Anton Emmanuel, consultant gastroenterologist at University College Hospital in London, estimated that it takes 2-3 hours for a 600 calorie roast dinner to be broken down in the stomach before moving on through the small intestine, colon and eventually being excreted around 24 hours later.

Constantly bombarding our stomachs with food so frequently will inevitably lead to the digestive system struggling to keep up, food being backed up, and our gut health being badly affected as a result.   All of this often results in common problems today such as constipation, wind, heartburn, and Gastroesophageal Reflux Disease (GERD).

#5 Spend less time on the toilet pan.

Quite often those people eating smaller meals will consume a considerably higher number of calories than is necessary to keep building muscle mass. Yep, more calories from good food sources, combined with proper weight training, does equal more muscle mass. It also equals more time in the bathroom when you overdo it so much.

Life's too short to be sitting on the toilet pan...straining...and wiping your ass 79 times per week! I spent 10 miserable years being a slave to my diet, and falling off and on the wagon trying to stick to six meals per day. I hated it but persisted because I thought it was the only way to maintain muscle.

It's not.

CHECKLIST

- Eating 6 or more small meals per day is not necessary for building muscle and keeping fat levels low.

- Meal frequency is a "matter of personal preference" – as long as sufficient calories and nutrients are being taken in over the course of the day.

- Taking longer stretches between meals helps optimise the master hormone leptin and insulin sensitivity, which makes the body more efficient at burning fat and building muscle.

- Eating in a normal fashion, i.e. 3-4 meals per day, rather than the typical bodybuilder approach has several benefits such as easing the strain on your digestive system and avoiding constant food prepping.

Chapter 2

The 7 Golden Rules Of Clean Eating

Eating clean all the time is a pain in the ass. I get it. That's exactly why I always recommend eating as healthy as possible Monday-Friday and then loosening up a little at the weekend...without going too nuts.

Eating 'clean' in the broadest sense means reducing the following as much as possible in your diet: ready meals, takeaways, sugary drinks and foods, and generally all processed junk. It also means staying well hydrated and making sure you're getting enough vitamins and minerals to give your body the right tools to keep you healthy and to support your strength training goals.

You could train like Rocky Balboa in the gym, but if your nutrition sucks then you're going to get nowhere. At the same time, you don't have to go to other extremes and follow a super strict diet to get in great shape and stay healthy. That'll only make you miserable and you'll eventually go on the rebound and end up on a 17 day junk food bender!

Seriously, if you want to make positive changes and get real results from your efforts in the gym then pay attention to the following Golden Rules of Clean Eating. Some of them may be stating the obvious, some might be completely new concepts to you. No matter where you're at health and fitness wise, these 7 steps will guide you towards great results.

If your diet hasn't been the best and you've got plenty of work to do, then here's a tip: introduce one positive habit per week. This is what I do with all clients who join my online personal training program. If we try to change everything at once it becomes overwhelming and makes you want to quit. If we focus on one positive habit per week, i.e. ditch fizzy drinks and replace them with water, then we can build upon each one and ultimately get awesome results at the end of the 10 week program.

Eat Clean Following These 7 Golden Guidelines

#1 Green is great

This means eating more vegetables and fruit. Stating the obvious here I know, but let's be honest - most of us don't eat nearly enough fruit and veg. Four or five servings per day is recommended to provide vitamins, minerals and a healthy source of carbohydrates. Try and include them with every meal.

#2 The white stuff ain't so great...

I'm talking about refined sugar. Excess sugar in our diets makes us fat and sick. Natural sugars from sweet fruits – yes. Fizzy drinks - complete no-no. We'll go into the problems of too much sugar in your diet, along with my tips and tricks to reduce it, in much more detail later.

#3 Cook fresh as much as possible

When buying the ingredients and preparing food yourself you know exactly what's going into your meals. No dodgy additives on the menu! I recommend investing in a vegetable steamer and blender. These are the two must haves in my kitchen. The steamer helps cook your vegetables lightly so that they retain their goodness. Boiling for too long, and even worse microwaving, remove the vitamins, minerals and enzymes from plant foods. Meanwhile, a blender is essential for making healthy protein shakes, either for breakfast or post-workout.

#4 Drink plenty of water

Men should shoot for around 3 litres per day, with women going for around 2.5 litres. Medics estimate that more than half of Americans are chronically dehydrated and this can lead to a multitude of health problems including headaches, weight gain, fatigue, joint pain and high blood pressure.

Weight training also causes water loss through sweating and, with our muscles being made up of 79% water, we require extra h2o to recover properly following a workout. Buy a sports water bottle and take it everywhere with you. To work, to the gym, when out walking the dog.

Get into the habit of having water handy and staying hydrated. We're also usually dehydrated in the morning after sweating in our sleep. I drink a pint of warm water with the juice from half a lemon when I wake up as this improves digestion, boosts your immune system, cleanses your body, and reduces inflammation.

#5 Beware of the long ingredients list

You'll have heard the "saying too many cook spoil the broth". Well, too many ingredients usually spoil the food. If the ingredients list on the packaging is long this generally means the food has been filled with too many chemical flavourings, preservatives and additives, and is likely to be processed to the point where there is little nutritional value.

When you start seeing too many weird words you can barely pronounce then steer clear. Here are a few examples...Butylated Hydroxyl-anisole', Monosodium Glutamate, Propyl P-hydroxybenzoate. Say what?

#6 Limit salt

Usually listed as 'sodium' on packaging, be careful that there's not too much in what you're eating. The recommended daily allowance of salt is 6g – one teaspoon – per day to avoid health issues like high blood pressure.

#7 Ditch the microwave

Microwaves zap the life out of your food, robbing it of digestive enzymes, vitamins and minerals. Most pre-packaged ready meals for the microwave often have little nutritional value in the first place compared to a meal cooked with fresh ingredients.

And 7 Ways To Help You Stay On Track...

#1 Avoid the booze

Okay we know alcohol is bad for us, but so is all the junk food we eat afterwards. Hangovers lower our blood sugar, make us feel terrible...and we usually turn to the unhealthiest foods to try and feel better. Hungover people naturally crave sugar, fat and simple carbs as a quick way to raise their blood sugar levels. If you're getting on a wee bit like me, then you'll know that the hangovers don't hang around for one day any more!

#2 Cook double the amount of food for dinner

Then have another serving for lunch the next day. This is an easy healthy habit to get into. Cooking freshly-made healthy dinners regularly at home is the way forward for eating clean – and you can kill two birds with one stone by cooking plenty and munching on the rest for lunch the following day.

#3 Don't buy in junk food

Let's be honest, if there's a choice between the good and bad stuff in our cupboards we'll probably go straight for the chocolate, biscuits, potato chips etc first. If they're within easy reach then they're going to get devoured at some point. Just remove temptation by completely bodyswerving them at the supermarket. Buy in plenty of vegetables and fruit, and stock up on healthy snacks such as packets of nuts and raisins, hummus, and oatcakes and natural unsweetened peanut butter.

#4 Don't hit that 'snooze' button too many times

If you're always out of bed late and rush around in the morning then your diet will always suffer. It's hard eating clean when you've only got 30 minutes to get showered, dressed, brush your teeth, get to work...and then think about filling your belly. Set the alarm a bit earlier than normal, fly out of bed, make yourself a delicious dish, and start the day as you mean to go on.

#5 Get breakfast and lunch ready the night before

Here's another way to make sure you don't grab a takeaway breakfast or eat junk on the run...make a healthy breakfast shake the night before. I mentioned earlier that a blender is a must have item in my kitchen and one could improve your diet big time too.

My book *Meal Prep: 50 Simple Recipes For Health & Fitness Nuts* includes 10 tasty shake recipes that I always mix up throughout the week. You could also just Google 'healthy smoothie recipes' or 'clean eating smoothie' to find plenty of shake ideas online. You can then grab the shaker as you run out the door and drink that on the way to work, rather than swinging past a fast food drive thru for a greasy breakfast.

#6 Think about how crappy you'll feel afterwards

When you're drawn towards a mega munch of treats, sweets and fast food, then focus on how you'll feel afterwards. How do you usually feel <u>after</u> a splurge when you've been trying to eat clean? The guilt usually kicks in pretty quickly, doesn't it? And there's a fair chance you'll feel bloated, tired, maybe even a bit sick after a large fast food meal. When you're struggling with the temptation of junk food, first focus on this familiar not-so-good feeling that usually occurs after you go off the rails. It can help you stay on track.

#7 Cut yourself a bit of slack at the weekend

As I mentioned earlier in this chapter, focus on eating super clean Monday-Friday and then cut yourself a bit of slack at the weekend. Making the right food choices consistently is essential, but don't treat eating and nutrition like some sort of military exercise. It'll never work – as most fad diets prove in the long run. You'll only end up back at square one.

Get stuck into your favourite takeaway meal on a Saturday night with some wine. Or popcorn and some chocolate at the cinema. As long as you don't go overboard, you'll still be able to make progress in your health and fitness goals.

CHECKLIST

- The 7 Golden Rules Of Clean Eating in a nutshell:

- Eat more vegetables and fruit.

- Cut right down on refined sugar, no more than 35g per day.

- Cook fresh as much as possible.

- Limit salt to no more than 6g per day.

- Drink 2.5 to 3 litres of water per day (ideally include a pint with fresh lemon juice in that too).

- Beware of foods with too many dodgy additives and preservatives, the names of which you can barely pronounce.

- Ditch the microwave...it zaps the goodness out of your food.

- And 7 ways to stay on track with clean eating...also in a nutshell:

- Avoid boozing as much as you can...it's only going to turn you into a junk eating monster.

- Make double the amount of food when cooking a home-made dinner – then have another serving for lunch the next day.

- Simply bodyswerve the junk food at the supermarket – because if it's in your cupboard you'll likely choose that before the healthy foods.

- Get up bright and early so you're not rushing around in the morning and have time to make a healthy breakfast and lunch.

- Alternatively, make a healthy breakfast shake the night before, put it in a shaker and then grab it on your way out the door the next day.

- Think hard about how crappy you'll feel after your junk food splurge – the more you do it the more it'll put you off.

- Eat clean Monday-Friday and cut yourself some slack at the weekend for some treats.

Chapter 3:

The 'Poison' In Our Diets

Are you struggling to lose the flab around your waist?

...annoyed at the lack of muscle definition?

...fed up eating tasteless 'low fat' foods – while not actually losing much fat?

...do you lack energy and catch every cold, infection, virus that is floating around?

Cutting back on sugar might well be the answer to your problems. Too much refined sugar on a daily basis will play havoc with your body – and prove to be a roadblock to getting in great shape and achieving optimal health. In fact, it's often considered a POISON to the body. Rewind to 1957 and Dr William Coda Martin first classified refined sugar as a poison because it is depleted of its life forces, vitamins and minerals when processed from sugar cane plants.

He said: "What is left consists of pure, refined carbohydrates. The body cannot utilise this refined starch and carbohydrate unless the depleted proteins, vitamins and minerals are present."

Fast forward to 1972, British physician and endocrinologist John Yudkin wrote the book *Pure, White and Deadly* warning of a health disaster due to the increase in consumption of sugar in our Western diets. And these days...

- Refined sugar contributes to around 35 million deaths around the world, according to researchers at the University of California. They commented in the journal Nature that it should be considered as toxic as tobacco and alcohol.

- Cancer, heart disease, diabetes, metabolic syndrome and a multitude of other diseases have been strongly linked with over-consumption of refined sugar.

- Childhood obesity is at record levels in the US, UK and in many countries across Europe where processed, junk foods fill most space on supermarket shelves.

- The UK government came under more pressure in October 2005 to introduce a 'sugar tax' due to its links with obesity and links to illnesses such as diabetes. This came after new stats show that one in five children in the UK are obese by the time they leave primary school.

- In the US, the number of people who had diabetes due to chronic blood sugar issues saw an "alarming" rise from 26 million in 2010 to 29 million in 2014, according to the Centers for Disease Control and Prevention.

Think I've made my point. Not only is sugar directly linked to diseases such as cancer and heart disease, it weakens the immune system and robs your body of essential vitamins and minerals needed for a strong, healthy body.

How Excess Sugar Makes Us Fat

Too much glucose is the first issue. Whenever we fill our bodies with too much fuel, which is very easy with high sugar foods, the liver runs out of storage capacity. The excess sugar is then converted into fatty acids and is then returned to the bloodstream. This is then stored as bodyfat in your belly, hips, chest...and generally most places you don't want it.

The second issue is excess insulin. Insulin is a key hormone in the body, and is released in high amounts whenever you eat or drink a "simple" carbohydrate, which includes the likes of white bread, white rice, baked white potato, bagels, croissants, cornflakes, cake, sugary drinks, beer, and anything that has high fructose corn syrup on the nutritional label.

When insulin levels are spiked the body's fat burning process is shut down so that the sugar that's just been consumed can be used for energy straight away. Sugar is shuttled into your muscles but, as soon as the muscle energy stores are full, the excess sugars are converted and stored as bodyfat. There are many ways you can drastically cut back on sugar in your diet and I'll share 10 simple ways you can start doing so today. First, here's a quick breakdown of different types of sugar.

- Sucrose – comes mainly from sugar cane or sugar beets.

- High fructose corn syrup (HFCS) – not technically a sugar, it is a liquid sweetener made from corn introduced to our diets in the 1970's.

- Fructose, maltose and dextrose – comes from fruits and starchy plants.

- Lactose – comes from dairy products.

Sugars consumed in large amounts contribute to obesity and disease, but the first two above are the real problem. Cane plants are stripped of all vitamins and minerals when refined to make common white sugar. In this state, it is considered toxic to the body by medical experts. Meanwhile, HFCS is an industrial food product which is far from natural.

The American Heart Association recommends that 37.5 grams (around 7 teaspoons) of added sugar is the daily limit for men, while 25g (around 5 teaspoons) is enough for women. One 330ml can of Coke contains 35 grams alone. Be aware that there's likely too much sugar in your foods if sugar is listed close to the top of the ingredients list. Also, sugar is not always listed as sugar. Look out for the names of its man-made dodgy cousins including high fructose corn syrup, dried cane syrup and brown rice syrup. If there are several of them in the one food item then I'd steer clear.

10 Simple Steps To Reduce Sugar In Your Diet

#1 One lump, not two

Have one sugar in your tea or coffee instead of two. Then cut back on the number of cups of tea/coffee you have every day...and gradually wean yourself off the sugar.

#2 Super Stevia

Even better, use Stevia. It is a 100% natural zero calorie sweetener with numerous health benefits. Studies have shown that Stevia can actually reduce blood pressure and fight type II diabetes.

#3 Go herbal

Try out herbal teas instead of tea, coffee or soda. Herbal teas are awesome, with lots of varieties that are full of flavour and decaffeinated too.

#4 Let the fizzy drinks fizzle out.

If you drink juice/soda throughout the day gradually cut back by swapping some for a cup of water instead. Wean yourself off the fizzy drinks gradually by replacing it with water instead.

#5 Change up your breakfast.

Do you eat cereal for breakfast? Most have high levels of sugar (Up to three teaspoons per small 30g bowl). So why not swap cereal for porridge or wholegrain toast with scrambled eggs?

#6 Ditch the desserts.

If you have desserts after dinner or chocolate most nights then gradually cut that out one day at a time.

#7 Add spices to your foods.

Cinnamon, ginger, nutmeg and cardamom will naturally sweeten your foods and reduce cravings for sugar.

#8 Don't buy sugary snacks.

The cravings will come and go for chocolate and other sweet foods, but if you don't have these snacks within easy reach in your house or work office then you will be able to cut down on sugar intake.

#9 Have a piece of fruit instead.

This can help satisfy sugar cravings and the natural sugars fruit contain are healthier than refined sugars.

#10 Read the labels.

Sugar is not always listed as sugar. Look out for names including high fructose corn syrup (remember than one?), dried cane syrup, sucrose and brown rice syrup. These can all be listed as separately on ingredients lists, and if the names are listed close to the top there is probably a considerable amount of sugar in the food.

Did the sugar message get through? Was all the chat about cancer, heart disease, diabetes and general doom as delightful and uplifting as I intended? Good - job done. Let's be honest, you (probably) won't drop dead after the next king size Mars bar you eat. But if you want to be healthy and are serious about getting in good shape then cutting out as much sugar as possible is a massive step.

Remember, excess sugar turns to fat – and both refined sugar and high fructose corn syrup are the worst offenders. Doesn't mean that you don't have to give up treats forever. Just follow the 10 steps above and gradually cut back your sugar intake overall.

CHECKLIST

- Refined sugar is considered a poison in many medical circles and has been directly linked to various killer diseases including diabetes, cancer and heart disease.

- Glucose overload from too much sugar results in the liver converting it into fatty acids. These are then returned to the bloodstream and stored as bodyfat.

- Excess sugar also causes our insulin levels to spike and, when our muscle energy stores are full, it is also stored as bodyfat.

- Look out for other forms of man-made sugars listed as high fructose corn syrup, dried cane syrup and brown rice syrup on food labels. Steer clear if there are several of these names on the packaging.

- Choose some, or all, of these options to reduce your sugar intake:

- Cut down on the sugar in your tea or coffee.

- Better yet, drink herbal teas.

- Choose natural sweetener Stevia instead of sugar.

- Ditch desserts after dinner.

- Replace fizzy drinks with water.

- Add spices to your foods for more flavouring.

- Don't buy in sugary snacks, there are healthier alternatives like fruit.

Read food labels and keep an eye out for high sugar content.

Chapter 4:

Making The Right Food Choices

Building muscle is not all about how much protein you eat. Losing fat is not about how much fat you eat. And carbohydrates are not all bad, despite all sorts of new 'low carb' or 'carb cycling' diets we hear about these days.

Diet and nutrition can get crazily complicated in the health and fitness industry. Fad diets, calorie counting, macronutrients calculations and fancy supplements. But the bottom line is that you won't gain lean muscle or be able to strip fat effectively if you don't get the basics of making correct food choices right. Our macronutrients are of course split into three categories: protein, carbs and fats. Each macronutrient can also be split into two more groups...the good guys and the bad guys.

Yep, the *sources* of your carbs, protein and fat are what's most important. Brown rice is high in carbs...but so is white bread. Deep fried chicken is high in protein and fat...so are almonds. Which will you choose? Let's take each of the three macronutrients and sort the good from the bad.

Carbohydrates

Carbs are the body's main source of fuel and it's a straight up battle between complex (the good guys) and simple (bad) carbs. Complex carbohydrates are unprocessed and contain the fiber found naturally in the food, while refined carbs have been processed and had the natural fiber stripped out.

Simple carbohydrates are made up of easy to digest sugars with little nutritional value for your body. The higher in sugar, the worse the carbohydrate is for you. Obviously cookies, sweets and desserts are among the worst offenders – but you can still enjoy them occasionally.

A much better option is for your daily intake to be made primarily made up of complex carbohydrates. Dietitians and nutritionists compare carbohydrate foods based on their glycemic index. This basically refers to how quickly and how high your blood sugar will rise after eating carbohydrates. Lower glycemic foods are healthier and most, but not all, complex carbs fall into this category.

The Goodfellas: sources of complex carbs include: vegetables, fruits, wholegrains, brown rice, beans, legumes, nuts and seeds. Fill up on these.

The Bad Guys: common simple carbohydrate foods include: cakes and cookies, pastries and desserts, white breads, white pasta, white rice. Limit these.

Protein

Protein's main role is for tissue growth and repair. Forget building muscle without a decent supply of protein. But how much protein do we need exactly? That's something we'll delve deeper into later. First, let's break protein down. Protein is made up of 'amino acids', which are the building blocks of the body for repairing and developing muscle. They also play a role in energy, weight loss, and brain function. Of the 20 amino acids, there are nine 'essential' ones, which the human body cannot produce.

What should be on the menu to build muscle? Food sources considered 'complete proteins' – meaning they contain all nine essential amino acids - or a combination of 'incomplete proteins' to ensure you cover all bases. Complete proteins are primarily animal-based foods and a few plant-based sources. These include: meat, poultry, fish, dairy products, eggs, quinoa, buckwheat, hemp seeds.

Have you Googled those last two already? No, they're not on my shopping list either. And don't panic if you're a vegetarian or vegan. You can still grab all essential amino acids and build muscle by feasting on a variety of incomplete protein sources including nuts, seeds, grains and vegetables. There are also some awesome plant-based protein supplements, such as brown rice protein and vegan blend protein, that I switched to years ago.

Personally, I avoid red meat and don't eat much animal protein at all, apart from chicken 3-4 days per week. My body finds it harder to digest meat and I believe there's truth in the arguments that too much animal protein is bad for our health. I'm not trying to convince you either way, I'll leave it up to you to do your own research.

Fats

Fat clogs your arteries. Fat makes you fat. Fat causes obesity. Fat started World War Two...I reckon fat gets a pretty bad rap. For decades the medical establishment had us believe that fat is at the root cause of our health problems. *'Eat a low fat diet and you will lose weight,'* they told us. *'Cut down on fat for better health,'* they promised.

Fact: The 'low fat' diet was first recommended to Americans back in 1977 – yet obesity has more than doubled since then.

Fact: The standard Mediterranean diet is as high as 40% fat, yet research has shown it cuts the risk of heart disease and strokes by around a third.

Fact: Eating those Satanic saturated fats, that we have been told we must avoid, is the best way to reduce a substance called lipoprotein – which is strongly linked to heart disease.

Just like carbs, there are good guys and bad guys when it comes to fat. There are four main types of fat: saturated (good), monounsaturated (good), polyunsaturated (okay, but when heated we have a problem) and trans-fats (bad).

Here's how I sum the whole situation up:

- Saturated fats are better for us than we were led to believe.

- Trans-fats (aka man-made ones) are to be avoided like the plague.

- Monounsaturated are good for us.

- Polyunsaturated fats are okay in moderation.

<u>The Goodfellas</u>: fish, unrefined animal fat, plant foods such as nuts, seeds, olives and avocados, eggs and dairy, olive oil, coconut oil etc. Get stuck into these.

<u>The Bad Guys</u>: fried foods, baked goods, margarine, and processed snack foods. I've also lumped vegetable oils (such as sunflower, corn, canola etc) in with the bad guys, but there is still debate about whether or not they're good for us. I err on the side of caution. Limit or eliminate these.

"Aren't saturated fats bad for us?...."

I can hear some readers saying this already. There's still plenty of debate over saturated fats, but it seems health experts are finally catching up to the idea that added sugars are public enemy #1, with dodgy man-made <u>trans-fats</u> (used in the likes of vegetable oil and margarine) also culpable. Plenty of leading medical researchers and top health and fitness experts, including the hugely-respected Charles Poliquin and Mark Sisson, have long argued the case that saturated fats are not only good for us, but they play some really important roles in the body.

Mark Sisson, of Mark's Daily Apple, recommends saturated fats in animal products and the likes of extra virgin olive oil as part of a healthy diet. He often writes about their importance in immune function, enhancing calcium absorption and providing fat soluble vitamins. The late Mary Enig PHd, nutritionist and researcher, had been screaming about how we had it all wrong on saturated fats for years. She spent decades studying the role of fats in the diet and disputed the widely held medical views that high levels of saturated fats caused heart disease.

Enig, who was awarded Master of the American College of Nutrition, argued that foods high in natural saturated fats, such as butter & coconut oil, are *beneficial* for heart health. *She wrote: "The much-maligned saturated fats—which Americans are trying to avoid—are not the cause of our modern diseases. In fact, they play many important roles in the body chemistry. The scientific evidence, honestly evaluated, does not support the assertion that 'artery-clogging' saturated fats cause heart disease."*

The American Heart Association still advises us to limit saturated fats, arguing that studies have shown it increases level of 'bad' cholesterol. Some other medical experts still believe too much saturated fat contributes to heart disease. I'm in the pro-saturated fat camp and reckon fats make up around 30%-40% of my diet. My main sources are butter, nuts and coconut milk.

Eating For Your Body Type

Food provides us with fuel and the nutrients needed for repair, growth and development. So how much protein, carbs and fats should someone involved in strength training be taking in to gain lean muscle and keep bodyfat low? The Institute of Medicine calculated an acceptable macronutrient distribution range for active people as: carbohydrate (45%-65%), protein (10%-35%), and fat (20%-35%).

Our bodies are different so there's no perfect ratio of macronutrients that applies to everyone, but by figuring out our body type we can get a fair idea of how to mix up our carbs, protein and fat. *Ectomorph, mesomorph* and *endomorph* body types each have different metabolic rates and hormonal responses to food. I was a 100% ectomorph (aka super skinny) before I took up weight training, but I'd say I'm more between ectomorph and mesomorph now that I've managed to gain and retain muscle mass due to years of training.

Ectomorph

This is the 'hard gainer' body type. Naturally slimmer people who have a faster metabolism and a higher tolerance for carbs. They can eat more junk food than most and generally get away with it. Their typical macronutrients split could be: carbs 55%, protein 25%, fats 20%.

Mesomorph

The people skinny and heavier dudes love to hate. They have a naturally athletic physique with more muscle mass and seem to get in great shape with less effort. Moderate carbs with higher ratio of protein and fats. Typical ratio would be: carbs 45%, protein 35%, fats 20%.

Endomorph

People with these body types pack on muscle with ease, but have a bigger, rounder frame and can struggle to lose weight. Their diet should have fewer carbs, with more protein and healthy fats. Typical ratio − carbs − 35%, protein − 35%, fats − 30%.

These are just averages and the ratios can be adjusted depending on the particular goal at the time. For example, an endomorph who wants to lose weight might cut carbs down further to 10-15%, bump up the number of protein foods, and add a few more healthy fat food sources. Or a mesomorph, who is neither fat nor thin but is looking to develop a six pack, might also cut carbs so that the body turns to fat stores for energy.

Whatever category you fall into, or if you're split between two, adjust your protein, carbs and fats to suit. If you're overweight and have a bigger frame, it would make sense to lower your carbs intake, while if you are too skinny you can take in more regularly to help add on some weight.

- Carbohydrates: more of the 'complex' variety, less of the 'simple' ones. Fill up on vegetables, fruits, wholegrains, brown rice, beans, legumes etc.

- Protein: meat, poultry, fish, dairy products, eggs and plant-based foods such as quinoa, buckwheat and hemp seeds are all good sources.

- Fat: avoid trans-fats (fried foods, margarine etc) as much as you can. Instead, get your fat fill from fish, unrefined animal fat, coconut oil, olive oil, plant foods such as nuts, seeds, olives and avocados, eggs and dairy.

CHECKLIST

- Carbohydrates are the body's main source of energy and are split into two types: 'complex' (the good guys) and 'simple' (the bad guys).

- Best carbohydrate sources: vegetables, fruits, wholegrains, brown rice, beans, legumes, nuts and seeds. Fill up on these.

- Worst carbohydrate sources: cakes and cookies, pastries and desserts, white breads, white pasta, white rice. Limit these.

- Protein builds muscle as one of its main roles is tissue repair and growth. Protein is made up amino acids which complete this process.

- Excellent protein sources: meat, poultry, fish, dairy products, eggs, quinoa, nuts, seeds, plant-based protein powder supplements.

- Not all fats are bad for us and, despite years of misinformation about saturated fat being unhealthy, it's argued now that saturated fat plays important roles in our bodies such as boosting the immune system, the manufacture of hormones and strengthening bones.

- Excellent fat sources: fish, unrefined animal fat, plant foods such as nuts, seeds, olives and avocados, eggs and dairy, olive oil, coconut oil.

- Fat sources to avoid: fried foods such as fries, crisps, cakes, margarine, processed snack foods, vegetable oils such as sunflower, corn, and canola.

- The 'ectomorph' naturally slimmer body type has a higher metabolism and a higher tolerance for carbs. Their typical macronutrients split would be around: carbs 55%, protein 25%, fats 20%.

- The 'mesomorph', aka naturally athletic body type, would eat roughly around: carbs 45%, protein 35%, fats 20%.

- The 'endomorph' bigger, rounder frame which adds muscle easily should have fewer carbs. Their typical ratio would be around: carbs – 35%, protein – 35%, fats – 30%.

Chapter 5:

How To Break Unhealthy Eating Habits

Every time a visitor walks into my living room these days they give me a funny look.

They gaze into the far corner of the room, try to figure out what's not right, and then it hits them about 7 seconds later. (I've been timing it).

"Where's your TV?" one friend after another asks. The TV stand is sitting there. The DVDs are still piled up neatly underneath, and the family photos are where they always sat too. But the big 50 inch TV that once took up a chunk of the room? It has been relegated to the floor of the spare bedroom that I barely go in.

Why? Because it was a huge distraction and it kept putting me off course as I tried to finish writing this book. Watching the weekend's UFC fights on the TV - or sitting down to concentrate and write? The TV would win. Watching three consecutive episodes of Animal Planet - or sitting down at my laptop to write more of the book? You guessed it, the TV would win again.

I realised that the only way to resist temptation and get on with some real work was to remove the "reward" of watching TV. There were so many wires hooked up to the TV, and carrying it all the way upstairs was a bit of a workout. Every time I contemplate watching the TV now I think of all the hassle it would take to bring it back downstairs, hook it all up again etc.

My clever productivity tactic worked - job done. My clients have successfully applied similar tactics to getting their diet on track. You can too.

Alan, one of my former clients, not only watched too much TV. He ate too much chocolate while doing it and, although he felt guilty as hell afterwards, he was hooked. He told me it was the same routine every day: eat dinner, wash the dishes, put the kettle on, and then grab a bar of chocolate from the cupboard next to the sink.

Sweet treats after dinner had become a bad habit. It almost became as routine as brushing his teeth every morning. I'm always telling my clients to lay off the sugar – but willpower wasn't going to be enough.

I explained to Alan that we had to remove the "reward" in this scenario for him to get anywhere. If we didn't he had no chance of kicking this unhealthy habit and improving his diet.

This is exactly the type of approach I recommend you take to improve your diet and nutrition too. Gradually remove negative habits one at a time. Gradually replace them with positive habits one at a time.

There is a specific way to do this effectively and to understand how you can successfully achieve it, I'm going to explain how habits work.

How To Overcome Your Unhealthy Eating Habits

If you have a sweet tooth, or maybe drink too much booze on a Friday night, it's not quite as simple as feeling determined and saying: "I'm definitely going to cut back." Sure, you might stick to your guns for two or three days, but your willpower will likely wilt and you'll cave in…because eating or drinking this way has become an unhealthy habit. These habits form a program in your mind, and it's extremely difficult to deviate from that program.

Here's how a habit is formed: cue > routine > reward. It's like a loop scenario.

Stage 1

Cue/trigger - Alan finishes his dinner and immediately thinks of having a sweet treat afterwards.

Stage 2

Routine - Alan does the dishes, puts the kettle on, and then heads straight for the chocolate cupboard with a big smile on his face.

Stage 3

Reward – he munches his way through the chocolate like feeling all pleased with myself…again with a big cheesy grin on his face. (Then beats himself up afterwards for giving into temptation).

Here's another example of how it could apply to cutting back on alcohol. Another former client, Scott, would shop at Marks & Spencer specifically at weekends because they would do a special 'dining for two' meal deal. He'd basically get a really nice meal for two (their food is awesome) and a bottle of wine for just £10. He thought this was such good value that he started buying the meal deal every Friday night for him and his girlfriend.

Problem was, that one bottle of wine wasn't enough and he'd buy some more later. Next thing he knows he's lying in bed the next day with a stinking hangover, skips the gym, and then heads to McDonald's for junk food to try and feel better. Sound familiar?

When you properly look at this scenario you can see how it pans out in the habit loop.

Stage 1

Cue/trigger - it's late Friday afternoon and the thought pops into Scott's head that the Marks & Spencer meal deal starts again today. He always remembers because it's a habit by now.

Stage 2

Routine - he heads straight there to raid the shelves and grab a bottle of wine before all the good stuff is gone.

Stage 3

Reward - he enjoys the meal and the wine with his girlfriend...but doesn't enjoy the hangover the next day quite so much.

To break these unhealthy habits we need to break the habit loop. The best way to do that? <u>Remove the reward</u>.

Now you can see why my living room TV stand has no TV - and my mates think I'm a bit weird. Now you'll understand why Alan decided to stop buying chocolate at the supermarket to stock it all up in the kitchen cupboard. And you'll realise why Scott now orders a Chinese takeaway for a Friday night treat instead...because it's not a meal deal that comes with wine too.

Everyone has their unhealthy habits when it comes to diet and nutrition. Trying to eat clean all the time ain't easy work, let's be honest. But you can make steady progress if you take steps to break the habit loop.

Spend 10-15 mins thinking about how you could improve your diet and consider the cue > routine > reward scenario. Identify ways you could remove the rewards completely to keep yourself on the right track and eventually banish habits holding you back.

Change might not happen as quickly as you'd like and it isn't always easy. But with time and effort, virtually any habit can be reshaped.

Change Just One Habit At A Time

I've mentioned this elsewhere in the book, but it's always worth repeating: don't try to change everything at once. You'll end up feeling overwhelmed and not get very far. I recommend singling out one unhealthy habit you can replace with a positive one per week.

Anything you can do to cut back on sugar and alcohol is a good place to start. Maintain this habit, but then on week two choose another, and so on. These positive habits build, you gain momentum, and a month or so down the line you could see big changes in your health, bodyshape and even your confidence levels. Each time you stick to your positive habit you gain a little bit more self-esteem and respect yourself more. All the small things do matter and they add up to big results over time.

Chapter 6:

Calories

So here's the deal: I'm not going to bang on about calories and insist you start counting them at every meal, every day, every week. That would make life pretty annoying. And I don't want you turning into some sort of Rain Man mathematician as a side effect of trying to get in great shape.

BUT...I'm going to be straight up and tell you that calories are rather important when it comes to hitting your health and fitness goals. Bottom line is: if you don't take in enough calories you've got no chance of building muscle, and if you're trying to lose weight and develop lean muscle then you're going to have to be in a calorie deficit for a period.

A kilocalorie (kcal), better known as calorie, is a measure of the amount of energy in our food. It supplies our body with fuel to get through the day, our activities, our workouts etc. If we regularly take in more than we expend we gain weight – and vice versa. When clients first come to me and tell me their fitness goals, one of the first questions I ask them is: *"Do you know roughly how many calories you take in each day?"*

I've yet to meet a single client who does. And that's cool because who wants to be tracking numbers all the time when we're enjoying our food? But when we've got a particular fitness goal to hit it helps us get there much sooner when we know our calorie numbers. When you reach your ideal weight/size level you don't have to be as precise, but it's still really beneficial to know *roughly* how many calories you should be taking in on an average day, and a *fair idea* of how many calories are in your meals.

It's not as boring as it sounds because once you've been tracking calories for a little while, you soon learn roughly how much is in most of the common foods you eat. For me personally, I hover around 2,300-2,700 calories per day to maintain muscle and stay at the same weight. If I eat less than 2,000 calories per day for a week or more then I lose weight.

Most people looking for support from me are overweight and want to lose weight and develop muscle. We reduce their daily calories, along with a strength training program, to focus primarily on dropping the excess bodyfat. Then we'll make calorie adjustments and continue lifting weights to develop muscle. If a slim person comes to me saying they struggle to gain even a single pound of muscle, we'll bump up their calories along with implementing a weight training program consisting mainly of compound exercises.

A Simple Formula For Working Out Your Daily Calorie Requirements

How many calories we require each day depends on various factors including sex, age, height, weight, and activity levels. But without getting too complicated and trying to make it a perfect science, there's actually a simple calculation for figuring out roughly how many calories an average active person requires. How many calories should you be consuming? Do the math...

<u>Maintenance:</u>*Bodyweight in lbs x 15 = number of calories*

<u>Weight gain:</u>*Bodyweight in lbs x 17 = number of calories*

<u>Fat loss:</u>*Bodyweight in lbs x 12 = number of calories*

Therefore the sums for 160lb guy aiming to gain weight and size while building muscle would shoot for around 2,700-2,800 calories (160 x 17 = 2,720). Or a 170lb woman looking to lose fat would aim for around 2,000 calories per day (170 x 12 = 2,040).

These equations are effective guidelines for each goal will and keep you right when it comes to calories. But they aren't set in stone and can be adjusted slightly as you progress. For example, I'm a hard gainer who struggles to put on muscle mass. If I really wasn't seeing much progress after a few weeks I might actually increase multiplying my bodyweight from 17 to 18.

Someone determined to lose fat might multiply their bodyweight by 11 instead of 12 to reduce their calories a bit further. By adjusting calories as necessary, making the right food choices, and lifting weights regularly you'll be well on track to hitting your targets and seeing real changes in your body.

Building Muscle and Losing Fat - Simultaneously

Muscle gain and fat loss – at the same time. It can be done. We know we need sufficient calories to gain muscle and a calorie deficit for burning fat.

We also know now how to work out roughly how many calories we need based on our personal goals. Calories are key to everything going to plan...but we don't just get them from the food and drink that passes our lips that day. We can also turn to stored bodyfat - which are essentially stored calories – to fuel our workouts and muscle building efforts.

Whenever there's a calorie deficit the body will turn to fat stores for energy. If you're using that energy to lift heavy weights in the gym then we're getting 2 for the price of 1 here...losing excess fat in order to build muscle.

Going back to the example from earlier about the 170lb woman trying to lose fat. We worked out that she should be consuming around 2,000 calories per day to achieve this. Her maintenance calories including exercise should have been around 2,500. Where will her body get the missing 500 calories needed for energy and to build muscle? By burning bodyfat. There are roughly 3,500 calories in a pound of fat. 500 calories times 7 days amounts to 1 full pound of bodyfat being lost while fuelling muscle development.

A Top Tool For Tracking Calories...And Optimising Your Diet

The 'MyFitnessPal' app does everything – apart from shouting "don't eat that!!" – to optimise your diet and keep track of your calories. It's free to download on the iTunes and Android app stores and I use it with all my online personal training clients.

Calculating your calorie targets? Working out how much protein/carbs/fat you're taking in? Saving regular foods and recipes?

Even scanning the barcodes of your food packets? This amazing app does it all for you. It's straightforward to use and will help you hit your health and fitness goals more easily. There are also demonstration videos for the app on YouTube for anyone who finds using it a bit tricky at first.

CHECKLIST

- A kilocalorie (kcal), better known as calorie, is a measure of the amount of energy in our food. It supplies our body with fuel to get through the day, our activities, our workouts etc.

- If we regularly take in more calories than we expend we gain weight – and vice versa.

- You don't have to count every single calorie, but if your fitness goal is to lose weight or gain weight then you should have a fair idea of your average calories in and out each day.

- The simplified calorie formula:

- <u>Maintenance:</u>Bodyweight in lbs x 15 = number of calories

- <u>Weight gain:</u>Bodyweight in lbs x 17 = number of calories

- <u>Fat loss:</u>Bodyweight in lbs x 12 = number of calories

- Whenever there's a calorie deficit the body will turn to fat stores for energy. If you're using that energy to lift heavy weights in the gym then it's 2 for the price of 1...losing excess fat in order to build muscle.

- Want the simple answer to tracking calories and monitoring your nutrition? Download the MyFitnessPal app and set up a free account.

Chapter 7:

Do We Really Need ALL That Protein?

The world's gone a bit mental for protein. People who barely exercise are drinking protein shakes these days, you can buy Weetabix 'Protein' in the supermarket, and I'm pretty sure I saw a Protein Mars bar in a shop the other day. C'mon, seriously?

People who do strength training generally end up pretty obsessed by protein. Eggs for breakfast, chicken for dinner, protein shake straight after training. What goes with it...whether it's wholegrain bread, vegetables, pasta...is usually an after-thought. We're usually too busy trying to figure out yet another way to cook our chicken breast first.

But is it really necessary? Do we really need ALL that protein?

Turns out we don't – and it took me the best part of 15 years (and 4,093 cans of tuna) to realise it. That's why this entire chapter is dedicated to debunking the myth that you need massive amounts of protein to maintain or build muscle. This book cost less than the price of a tub of protein powder and if I'd known years ago what I know now I would have saved a fortune on food and supplements. This chapter alone could save you $$$$ too – and possibly even your health.

I've heard stories of personal trainers telling women to eat 180g, 200g or more of protein per day while doing strength training. These 125lbs women are loading up on eggs, bacon, whey protein shakes...struggling to get through it all each day to hit their protein targets. Then they're surprised when they're bloated, farting like mad, and are constantly constipated. Let's put that kind of protein intake into perspective....

Arnold Schwarzenegger, the world's greatest ever bodybuilder, weighing 220lbs, standing, 6ft 2 ins tall, only consumed around 150g of protein. This was when he was competing for the Mr Olympia title – which he won seven times. Meanwhile, these women are eating MORE protein than him - it doesn't make one bit of sense. We all know that protein builds muscle....but, again, do we really need ALL that protein?

I did a lengthy amount of research on this topic because, let's be honest, there's so much advice out there on diet, nutrition, supplements, macronutrients, micronutrients....that sometimes it makes you just wanna eat pizza and tell the health and fitness world to fuck off. I was really surprised about what I discovered and it appears that some protein myths that have been spouted by 'experts' and the multi-billion dollar protein supplement industry for decades.

You might choke on your protein shake while reading this but what if someone told you that....

- You could probably cut your protein intake by half – and still build and maintain muscle.

- One of the world's most famous bodybuilders only ate 60g of protein per day.

- An athlete who was consuming 300g of protein per day was shocked to discover most of it was going to waste...and he was developing worrying health problems as a result.

- Calories are a bigger factor when it comes to building muscle than you would believe.

- Our bodies can actually recycle amino acids themselves, meaning there is less need for a constant high supply of protein.

When it comes to building muscle and developing a strong, lean physique, the vast majority of experts in the health and fitness industry will tell us: "Eat more protein. Eat more protein...then have another plateful of protein." We're told to simply increase our protein numbers, train hard...and the muscle will come. The standard advice dished out by bodybuilders is: "You need 1g of protein per 1lb of bodyweight."

Some adverts in health and fitness magazines (which get paid megabucks for adverts by protein supplements companies funnily enough...) tell us we need as much as 300g or 400g to build maximum muscle. So while we're trying to cram in the equivalent of 10 x chicken breasts, or 12 cans of tuna, or 8 protein shakes, maybe it's worth asking who actually came up with these numbers anyway?

This more protein = more muscle idea seems too simplistic. Two very important factors are often ignored/forgotten about...

Protein **absorption** - a healthy digestive system can properly process the foods we eat to provide energy, extract the nutrients to nourish our cells, and help to build and repair muscle. Problem is, a high percentage of people living in the Western world <u>don't</u> have healthy digestive systems due to the processed junk that fills our supermarket shelves. The fact that the treatment of heartburn, constipation etc is a multi-billion dollar industry in America is proof of this. Many of us also live highly-stressed lives, and in times of stress our digestive system basically shuts down as our bodies go into 'fight or flight' mode. This means we don't break down food as we should - and certainly can't cope with ridiculous amounts of protein in those situations.

Secondly, the protein **source** is also an important factor. There are countless high protein foods we can choose from, but they are not all equal in nourishing the body and building muscle. For example, steak is one of the highest sources of protein and also contains a good dose of iron and creatine that you won't find in most other foods. It's hugely popular with bodybuilders - but takes up to 72 hours to be properly digested in the body.

It's not unusual for some bodybuilders to eat steak every other day in an attempt to keep building muscle. While the body is still processing the last one, along with other meals in between, it's looking highly likely that we're going to have some backing up of food. The body struggling to keep up is when digestive problems occur and toxins floating around in the body as a result can also lead to other health issues such as skin problems.

Is All That Extra Protein Going To Waste?

But how can we know for certain either way? How much of all that protein is actually being utilised by the body? <u>Not much</u> – is the answer from Dr Ellington Darden. After carrying out a unique two month-long protein study on himself back in 1970 and finding startling results,

Dr Darden insisted that *"the biggest misconception 20 years ago, and still the biggest misconception today"* is the idea that we need huge people lifting weight need a huge amount of protein to build and maintain muscle.

This isn't the opinion of just another "fitness expert". Dr Darden was honoured by the President's Council on Fitness, Sports and Nutrition as one of the top ten health leaders in the United States. Back in 1970, as a competitive athlete and bodybuilder for around 20 years he was consuming 380g of protein per day. Half of this came from protein powder and he was also popping all sorts of nutritional pills to aid his muscle growth.

That was until one of his colleagues, Dr Harold Schendel Professor in the Food and Nutrition Department at Florida State University, told him that was way too much protein and he was wasting his time. Determined to prove he was right, Dr Darden set up a detailed study on his own body. For two months, he kept precise records of his dietary intake, of energy expenditure, and his general well-being. All his urine was collected and analyzed by a graduate research team in nutrition science.

The results? The study showed his body was excreting large amounts of water soluble vitamins, proteins and other nutrients. As he had been consuming massive doses for years, his liver and kidneys had apparently grown excessively large to handle the influx of all these nutrients.

Why You Need Less Protein Than You Think

If you've been lifting weights for a while I'm guessing you're devouring tons of high protein foods like steak, chicken, eggs, whey protein shakes etc. We work so hard to build the muscle that we want to make sure we make the most gains afterwards. We even watch the clock every day to figure out when to guzzle the next protein shake or have our mid-morning snack. If we don't our gym efforts will go to waste, right?

The idea of reducing our protein intake – even on the advice of hugely respected experts like Dr Ellington Darden – terrifies most weightlifters (aka protein addicts) like you and me. Let's look at some of the main reasons why:

#1 The Fear That Cutting Down On Protein Will Result In Muscle Loss

This is without doubt the biggest worry. The standard advice from the health and fitness industry is more protein = more muscle, and so we keep increasing it as we get bigger and stronger. Here are three examples that completely debunk this theory.

<u>1</u> – Mike Mentzer was a bodybuilding champion who won the Mr Universe title in 1978 and in 1979 won the heavyweight class of the Mr Olympia competition...both with perfect 300 scores.

Mike's daily protein intake....60g per day. Yes, just 60g per day for a heavyweight competing athlete. Now I know genetics come into play with guys like Mike Mentzer but some weightlifters have his entire daily protein intake for breakfast alone. <u>Mike placed more emphasis on calories than excessive grams of protein.</u>

Before he died in 2001, Mike said: *"Protein requirements depend almost entirely on your bodyweight, not your level of physical activity, because it is not used as fuel as long as the body's energy supply is adequate. The rule of thumb is one gram of protein per day for every two pounds of bodyweight."*

Mike also insisted that buying expensive supplements was a waste of money because we can get what we need from a balanced diet which includes meat, fish or dairy products.

<u>2</u> – Dr Nick Delgado is a nutritional expert who tells us the same thing. He insists we require way less protein than we think – and also maintains that sufficient calories are more important. He follows a vegan diet and only eats around 60g of protein per day. In that case, you might imagine he's a bit of a weakling eh?

Afraid not, Dr Delgado holds a world strength endurance record in the Guinness Book of Records for pressing the most weight overhead in an hour (53,640 pounds!) Dr Delgado says that it's important we take in enough calories, arguing that a protein intake of between 45g and 75g is generous.

<u>3</u> – I mentioned earlier that even Arnold Schwarzenegger consumed around 150g of protein per day (around 0.7g per 1lb of bodyweight). This is still relatively small for a 220lb guy who was training hard for

the Mr Olympia world titles. Yet, I don't think anybody could argue with his results.

Also, a study was carried out in 2010 on 8 healthy men, who were each given infusions of amino acids (the building blocks of protein) over three hours. Protein synthesis increased with the influx of more amino acids – but then it began to decrease even though more amino acids were still being given. This suggests that bombarding the body with more protein does not necessarily mean more muscle.

#2 The Worry That It Will Lead To Too Much Weight Loss

Protein is not the body's primary fuel supply, carbohydrates are. By eating a sufficient amount of complex carbs and healthy fats too you can ensure the body's caloric needs are met. This helps maintain an ideal bodyweight, and has a protein sparing effect allowing you to develop muscle through strength training.

For 'hard-gainers' like myself who struggle to add a pound of weight (but can easily lose two or three after a weekend on the booze), it is a good move to focus on increasing healthy fats. Fat contains 9 calories per gram, while protein and carbs contain just 4 grams each. On your shopping list add more nut butters, coconut milk, coconut oil, butter, olive oil, avocados etc.

#3 The Fear Of Gaining Too Much Weight

The complete opposite to the worry above, but a genuine fear for people who have slimmed down by following a high protein diet and by training hard. Our bodies are all different in terms of composition, metabolism, how well we process some foods etc. BUT – if you reduce your excessive protein intake and still stick to a diet that is largely made up of whole foods (i.e. plenty fresh veg and fruit, whole grains, no processed junk) then it's very difficult to go wrong...particularly if you're also lifting heavy.

The Protein Scale For A Weightlifter

Okay, so there are plenty of different opinions about how much protein we need to maintain and build muscle. And we obviously know this varies based on bodyweight. But let's look at the scale based on the information and the people referred to in this article.

- World Health Organisation – 35g.

- Dr Nick Delgado, world strength endurance champion - 45g-75g.

- Mike Mentzer, former Mr Universe and Mr Olympia - 1g of protein per 2lbs of bodyweight.

- Arnold Schwarzenegger - 1g of protein per 2.2lbs of bodyweight.

- Standard bodybuilding community recommendation – 1g of protein per 1lb of bodyweight.

- Advice from some protein supplement companies – 300g-400g per day.

Starting at the bottom end...let's be honest, you would probably eat that much before lunchtime. The World Health Organisation is also giving recommendations for the average person, not someone who lifts weight regularly. Going to the other end of the scale, these figures of 300g-400g are crazy, needless amounts. Dr Ellington Darden's detailed two-month long study clearly showed that large amounts of protein goes to waste.

The standard bodybuilding advice is that we must eat 1g of protein per 1lb of bodyweight. This figure has been around for decades...yet we don't know who made it up and on what basis. Yet two of the finest bodybuilders the world has ever produced are telling us we only need HALF that amount. This advice from Arnie and Mike Mentzer lies slap bang in the middle of the scale and is what I would consider the most sensible.

My recommendation: **1g of protein per 2lbs of bodyweight** is an ideal target to aim for.....but, crucially, supported by a sufficient number of calories from complex carbohydrates and healthy fats.

Chapter 8:

The Importance Of Gut Health

As I sat staring at my computer screen I felt bloated, crappy, tired…and feared I'd need to run to the toilet to spew.

It was just after 4pm and I was supposed to be heading straight to the gym after work in an hour's time. "There's no way I'll be lifting much weight feeling like this", I said to myself.

This was my usual routine on gym training days. Breakfast before work, lunch finished by 1pm, and then a mid-afternoon protein shake to maintain my hard-earned muscle.

I thought that having the additional shake in between my lunch and my gym training session was a good idea. My stomach was telling me otherwise. It felt all hard and compacted; as if the pink sludgy shake had just solidified into a solid block at the pit of my stomach.

This was 10 years ago when I was working as a newspaper journalist. And like every good journalist does I decided to do some digging - on why I was feeling so ill. I followed a healthy diet, I lifted weights regularly, looked after my body…what was going on? Was I allergic to what I ate for lunch? Did I buy the wrong type of protein powder?

I began scrolling through online fitness forums looking for answers. I was thinking that maybe I should have adjusted my meal timing. Or that I was eating too many carbs and not enough protein? Then something caught me by surprise.

I noticed a post from a gym-goer who was saying he turned into a human farting machine every time he drank his protein shake. What caught my attention was the number of guys commenting underneath reporting similar stomach issues.

Feeling bloated. Feeling sick. Definitely not feeling fit, strong and healthy. That's exactly how I was feeling too, and seeing these comments online made me realise what was really going on in my belly.

My digestive system was still struggling to process the previous meal when I would pour a thick, sludgy, sweetened protein shake down my throat on top of it. Many people may get away with that for weeks, or months, at a time. I'd been doing this for years and to make matters worse my shakes were made with full fat milk. Milk is notoriously difficult for a section of society to digest properly because it contains lactose which some people cannot tolerate.

When my weight training journey began there had been a big focus on making the most of my hard gym efforts by eating healthy meals regularly, wolfing down as much protein as possible, and giving my body everything it needed to build muscle and keep bodyfat levels low.

What my body really needed was a break. My digestive system had effectively gone on strike after years of ramming meal after meal, shake after shake, and healthy snack after healthy snack down my throat. At one point my doctor diagnosed me with IBS and told me I'd need to take pills for the rest of my life.

I had a different diagnosis: I was suffering from Not-Giving-A-Fuck-About-My-Digestive-System-itis.

The prescription: learning all about what I was doing wrong and how to look after my guts in future.

What's the point trying to build muscle, get in great shape, and look amazing on the outside, if you feel terrible and start flushing your good health down the toilet?

Why bother counting the grams of protein in your meals when your body is struggling to make proper use of it all?

Why waste your money on sports supplements to try and enhance your body when what it really needs is some TLC for your guts.

The Digestive System: The Foundation of Good Health

A properly functioning digestive system is essential for good health. Training hard in the gym is only the first in a three part sequence. Lifting weights causes a low level of stress on the body, along with tiny tears on muscle fibres, and some strain on the joints.

Part two: our body is then screaming for nutrients to get to work on repairing the body and developing it. To be able to properly extract and utilise the nutrients from your food, the digestive system has got to be in good working order.

Part three: proper rest and recovery is needed, allowing the body to work through the night repairing itself and making full use of your earlier meals.

But what if something goes wrong in part two? What if your stomach also goes on strike? What if something breaks down in that complex factory of endless intestines, trillions of bacteria, enzymes, hydrochloric acid, bile…? What could possibly halt production in the factory? How could you fix it?

I'll answer these questions soon but first I want to give you a very basic rundown of how the digestive system works. It's a pretty complex subject and deserves a whole book to itself, but we're not here to get overly scientific and really geek out on things like bacteria and faeces. So I'll break it down as simply as possible.

Stage 1: The digestive process begins before you even put a forkful of food into your mouth. Just seeing and smelling food causes the brain to trigger the release of more saliva, which contains enzymes like amylase and lipase. That's why we're told to chew our food well because these enzymes help break our food down before it passes into our stomach.

Stage 2: Hydrochloric acid and enzymes are released in the stomach to break down our food into smaller parts and begin protein breakdown. Stomach acid also destroys the most harmful bacteria that may have been swallowed with your food or drink. But little nutrient absorption takes place at this point, this is an earlier dismantling phase of food into 'chyme'.

Stage 3: The chyme is then slowly squeezed down into the small intestine. This is where absorption begins and it can take between 4-8 hours for the chyme to travel the full length of the small intestine. In the first part of the small intestine, the duodenum, pancreatic juices are released containing bicarbonate to neutralize the acidic chyme and enzymes to break it down further for absorption. Bile is also released from the gallbladder to help process fats.

As the chyme moves through the small intestine most nutrients, such as magnesium, iron, zinc, water soluble vitamins, and amino acids, are absorbed.

Stage 4: The remaining chyme passes into the large intestine/colon for final processing. It absorbs remaining minerals like potassium and sodium, along with acids, gases and water in the chyme, leaving only our waste as faeces. It's in the large intestine where our body's good and bad bacteria lives. In this final stage of digestion, intestinal bacteria ferments carbohydrates that our bodies did not absorb properly, while disposing of enzymes, dead cells etc.

The Role Of Gut Bacteria

Aswell as playing a critical role in the final absorption of nutrients, an optimal balance of bacteria in the colon can prevent allergies, prevent yeast and pathogens from spreading in the gut, and fend off inflammatory bowel disease.

Your gut is made up of around 100 trillion of these microscopic bacteria - good guys and bad guys. The problems occur when the bad guys start taking over and things get out of balance. Too much bad bacteria in the gut can lead to a multitude of health problems, and will affect your body's absorption from foods.

Your gut flora can boost the immune system and protects against invaders in various ways. A healthy balance of gut bacteria strengthens the defences of the gut wall and competes with pathogens for space and food, leaving nothing for the bad guys. It also regulates inflammation and the inflammatory immune response in the body.

What Can Negatively Affect Your Gut Health

There are various factors, some of which may surprise you, that will mess with your digestion and overall absorption.

#1 Food intolerances and sensitivities

This is when certain foods cause an inflammatory reaction in the gut. Our bodies are all different and some people can tolerate certain foods, while in others it can trigger symptoms such as diarrhoea, stomach pain or headaches. The most common food intolerances are with dairy and gluten, but it's estimated that three in four people have some sort of food intolerance.

Consuming foods that your body doesn't tolerate well can lead to the intestinal lining becoming inflamed or damaged. This affects nutrient absorption and also triggers a negative immune system response.

#2 Too much stress

When we're overly stressed our body goes into 'fight or flight' mode and the digestive system effectively shuts down temporarily. The blood flow to your gut is affected and that's why you may get stomach upsets or feel rundown in times of heightened stress.

Good bacteria is also responsible for helping to signal the proper response to the brain to cope with elevated stressors so that the rest of the body isn't badly affected. But chronic stress can eat away at the good guys that, ironically, are trying to protect you from the effects of stress.

#3 Highly processed foods

Refined junk foods are bad for the body because they're often loaded with sugar, salt, chemical preservatives and additives, and synthetic and rancid fats. Studies have shown that processed foods, such as fast food takeaway meals, sweets and fizzy juice, can also have a detrimental effect on your immune system and gut health because the body struggles to cope with breaking it all down.

#4 Too much sugar

The typical Western diet includes way too much sugar and this has been increasingly linked to the overgrowth of bad bacteria in the colon and even gut inflammation. Scientists also believe the consumption of too much sugar may slow the transit time of food going through the gut. This can lead to various stomach issues including bloating and constipation.

#5 Antibiotics

You know those little pills the doctor gives you to kill off the bad guys making you sick? Well, they also kill off the good guys. Antibiotics play a major role in healthcare, but these drugs are also ruthless when it comes to your gut flora. A course of antibiotics could wipe out a substantial amount of your good bacteria, leaving your body out of balance. Fortunately, you can take steps to counter this and replace the bacteria you actually wanted to hang on to.

#6 Too much alcohol

Drinking excessively can disrupt the intestinal environment and negatively affect the balance of gut flora. Not only can alcohol abuse cause bad bacteria to flourish and take hold, it can also lead to gut permeability, which is also known as leaky gut syndrome. This problem results in undigested food particles breaking through the damaged intestinal wall and into the bloodstream, causing an inflammatory immune response.

How To Improve Gut Health

#1 Probiotics

Probiotics are live bacteria that are great for digestive health. These are often referred to as "good" or "helpful" bacteria because they keep your gut healthy. Probiotics are found in specific foods and they proliferate the good bacteria populating your large intestine. They also play an important role in strengthening the immune system.

Great sources of probiotics are foods like natural (unsweetened) yoghurt, sauerkraut, pickled foods, kefir, fermented vegetables. These typically can contain billions of beneficial bacteria such as acidophilus and lactobacillus, the most common probiotics found in yoghurt and fermented foods. These assist in absorbing nutrients and can help with IBS symptoms.

#2 Prebiotics

Similar name but not the same. Prebiotics are a type of fibre and act as food for probiotics, encouraging them to grow and improve your gut health further. Good sources of prebiotics include raw garlic, leeks, onions, bananas, and asparagus. Including those foods in your diet, along with rich probiotic sources, is a good step towards a healthier gut.

#3 Take steps to reduce stress

I explained above why too much ongoing stress is bad not only for your gut, but overall health. Do everything you can to look after your physical and mental wellbeing, whether that's taking long, relaxing baths, going for walks with the dog, meditating, or going for a stroll listening to your favourite music. Sounds pretty insignificant but I'd recommend taking these small steps every day to get away from pressure environments and simply put yourself first. Your gut will thank you for it.

Chapter 9:

The Mistake Of Following Typical Bodybuilding Advice

He's a health and fitness industry leader and has coached thousands of clients from across the world on improving their nutrition and training.

The Northern Irishman – currently based in Amsterdam – has featured in Men's Health, Women's Health, the BBC and was also a writer for the MyProtein website.

Introducing Ru Anderson, owner of Exceed Nutrition and author of best-selling book High Performance Living. I interviewed Ru and share his story here because it follows on perfectly from the previous chapter on the importance of looking after your digestive system.

A decade ago, Ru realised he was "destroying his health" by following the typical advice in fitness magazines and bodybuilding forums. It took him a while to discover that he'd neglected two important things in his mission for more muscle.

Ru's approach to training and nutrition has changed entirely since. He reveals why 8+ hours of sleep per night is now a top priority, along with looking after his gut health of course.

"I was overweight, felt pretty horrendous and my performance in day-to-day life wasn't much better…"

Not the kind of thing you'd expect to hear from a guy like Ru Anderson. He's in amazing shape – and has helped countless personal training clients to transform their bodies and health. But the fitness professional admits that he was damaging his health a decade ago because he went down the bodybuilding road.

Ru made the mistake of listening to the mainstream advice in fitness magazines and online forums. Dodgy diet tips, overtraining and crappy supplements all fully focused on muscle and size…

But with little thought towards digestion, energy levels and overall health.

Ru said: "In my mission to add large amounts of muscle, lean up, and build my strength, I forgot about two other major components: how I felt and how I performed.

"And I didn't realise how they would radically affect me. I was so focused on changing the outside of my body, that I neglected (and ignored) how I was feeling and performing on the inside.

"I was doing a lot of hard 'bodybuilding' training and following the typical magazine nutrition advice. The result? I got overweight, felt pretty horrendous and my performance in day-to-day life wasn't much better.

"I was constantly fatigued from the intense training, lacked concentration throughout the day, and had little energy left for any other activities. Aside from my dedicated 'gym time', I was pretty damn useless.

"To top it off, the mainstream nutrition advice I was being told to follow by magazines and forums was actually destroying my health, giving me IBS symptoms and skin issues like acne."

Ru added: "It was clear I had to find another way. So, armed with my new goal, I decided to study and experiment with a huge number of nutrition and training protocols.

"After throwing out the rubbish (which was most of it), I was left with a surprisingly powerful yet pretty simple set of principles. I've since gone on to prove them time and time again. These principles allow me and my clients to create and maintain healthy, lean, strong and energetic bodies.

"The biggest benefit from these changes is that I was able to achieve the body and health I had initially set out for."

Through his company Exceed Nutrition, Ru has coached many people on improving their nutrition, health and lifestyle. Men and women of all shapes, sizes and states of health have gone on to great success after introducing Ru's dietary principles and cutting out common mistakes.

Ru said: "A lot of my clients are motivated for change, which means they jump straight in and go 'all out' from the start. This usually leads to burning out and all of the extra effort is not usually so quickly rewarded. This can then result in a drop in motivation and interest.

"Changing your body can be a slow process, so trying to use every trick or strategy from the offset is not usually a good idea. So instead we start with the least amount of changes we need to achieve weekly results and progress."

Ru's Top 3 Tips for Looking, Feeling and Performing at Your Best

#1 Focus on recovery

"A big factor to bigger muscles and greater strength is the ability to fully recover from your training efforts. Train hard, but ensuring you can recover from it is key.

"Many magazines and programs can push your recovery abilities too far, because they have been created by athletes or those using assistance. Find a program that you can train hard with, but recover fast on."

#2 Focus on sleep

"Understanding the power of sleep and how to get as much high quality sleep as possible is one of the healthiest things you can do. We can all relate to how loss of sleep can take its toll on our energy, mood, decision-making and ability to handle stress.

"Sleep should therefore be your top priority. Many people try to sleep as little as possible, but just as exercise and nutrition are important to look and feel your best, so is sleep.

"No other activity delivers so many benefits with so little effort. Sleep has a direct correlation to the quality of your waking life. A must for me each night is 8+ hours, and I find most people do well on this too."

#3 Remove food sensitivities and intolerances

"In today's busy society, it's our lifestyles, nutrition and environment that hold us back and puts a negative strain on most of our body's systems. The digestive system is one of these systems.

"There is a strong argument from alternative medical practitioners that the food we eat is a frequently overlooked origin of disease. With a food allergy or sensitivity, the problematic food can set up a cascade of immune and chemical reactions in the body, usually within days (if not minutes) of ingestion.

"If this food is continually consumed over time, it can cause an on-going inflammatory reaction on the lining of the intestines, which can result in the lining becoming unhealthy.

"Our gut prevents dangerous toxins and compounds getting in whilst the foods and water we consume to enter the body. When our gut is not working optimally, or is in a state of distress, these dangerous compounds can enter our system, and the body will not fully absorb key nutrients from food.

"Basically, look after your gut in every way possible."

Chapter 10:

Pre-workout Nutrition

We all have the same gym pre-workout problem...

Trying to figure out exactly what the hell to eat/drink/gorge on for enough energy to get through a tough gym session and make the best progress possible. On one hand we want to feast on plenty of food for fuel. On the other we don't want it to leave us feeling like we need a nap afterwards!

"Load up on carbs for energy," they tell us. Have you tried the big plate of pasta mid-afternoon? Did you feel bloated like a balloon?

"Drink a meal replacement shake for extra calories," they said. Does that make you feel like a human slug by the time you start lifting weights?

Or the plain old banana that everyone tells you is a great source of energy. They're clearly bending the truth with that one. And don't get me started on those rubbish energy drinks. They contain ridiculously high amounts of sugar, all sorts of chemicals and additives, and if you'd like another reason not to drink them then Google "energy drinks deaths".

Fact is: nothing really cut it – until I came across 'The Two C's'. One natural supplement. One drink you probably have every day. Both beginning with the letter 'C'.

The Two 'C's: Coffee and Creatine

A plain cuppa black **coffee** and some **creatine** = an outrageously good combo for firing up your energy levels and boosting your performance in the gym. Taking these on an empty stomach ahead of a morning workout is highly effective for burning fat. This also sets the body up to be in a highly anabolic state when you have your post-workout meal.

I first heard about creatine around 15 years ago when I was still at college. I was out drinking on a summer's night at a local pub and I spotted a guy who was in my year at school. I hadn't seen him for a couple of years and the first thing I noticed was how big his arms and shoulders were. He had morphed into this muscley mutha and it didn't look like he had been taking anything dodgy like steroids. He was just in much better shape compared to last time I'd seen him.

Must admit, I remember feeling pretty gutted in that moment. I had been training pretty hard for around three years at that point and saw *some* gains, but looking at this dude was like a slap in the face waking me up. I figured that either I wasn't training hard enough – or I had just been going the wrong way about my weight training completely.

So I pulled him aside and – while trying not to sound like a jealous weirdo who had been eyeing up another guy's muscles at the pub – I asked: *"Mate, you're in great shape. You must be training constantly. What are you doing exactly?"*

It was then he told me he had been taking creatine as a pre-workout supplement, along with the same brand's protein powder post-workout....and had gained about 10lbs of muscle in a matter of months. It had always been a nightmare for me to gain just two or three pounds. So I was sold on this stuff already.

The next day I headed to the shop in Glasgow where my ex schoolmate bought his creatine. The creatine worked a treat. I put on around 6 or 7 pounds within the first couple of months and my strength went through the roof. I go through cycles of taking creatine now (two months on, one month off), but still get the same boost in power and performance in the gym 15 years later.

Creatine – The What, Why And How

Basic science behind creatine: it's an amino acid that's found in various foods and is also naturally produced in the body, helping to deliver energy to all cells, primarily muscles. Creatine increases the formation of ATP (adenosine triphosphate), which is the molecule that fuels life. ATP is where our cells get the energy to perform tasks. Essentially, more creatine = more ATP = more energy and power for workouts.

How it works: creatine has been proven to be effective in improving performance in weightlifters and other athletes. This is because it increases the body's ability to produce more energy rapidly, meaning you can train harder and for longer.

How to get more of it: beef and salmon are among the best food sources of creatine – but you would have to eat silly amounts to get the levels you need. That's why, since 1993, creatine has become a popular supplement in powder/capsules for athletes. There are several forms of this supplement but creatine *monohydrate* has been shown to be the most effective and is the most widely used.

The Benefits Of Supplementing With Creatine

As well as leading to an improvement in strength and an increased capacity for high intensity work, supplementing with creatine can reap various other benefits including:

- **Fuller muscles** – creatine enhances the volume of muscles. This is mainly achieved through increasing the fluid content of the muscles. It pulls more water in, giving them a fuller look.

- **Enhanced recovery** – a study on creatine supplementation was carried out in 2004 involving 34 men running a 30km race. Eighteen men used 20g of creatine mixed with maltodextrine per day for five days, while the others used only maltodextrine. Closely monitoring several markers of cell damage in both groups, researchers concluded: *"Creatine supplementation reduced cell damage and inflammation after an exhaustive intense race."*

- **Better brain function** – creatine supplementation can improve short term memory and also protect against neurological disorders, studies suggest. In 2003, a study was carried out on 45 young adults where they took 5g of creatine per day for six weeks, then took tests on memory performance and intelligence. Researchers concluded that *"creatine supplementation had a significant positive effect"*.

Is Supplementing With Creatine Safe?

First off, it's worth reminding that creatine is not a drug of any sort. It's a natural compound produced in the body and that can also be absorbed from various food sources. There have been scare stories over the years that prolonged use of creatine can cause kidney problems, but this has been disproven in countless studies. Other negative effects have also been highlighted, such as stomach cramps.

These supposed side effects are all well addressed in an article titled '*Six Side Effects Of Creatine: Myths Debunked*', which was published on Bodybuilding.com in November 2015. This well-researched, in-depth report is definitely worth a read if you have any concerns about taking creatine for the first time. The article underlines why it's a safe and effective supplement for healthy individuals and is backed up by 31 different studies.

- NOTE: People diagnosed with gout are advised not to take creatine as it will worsen the condition. If you have any health issues at all consult your doctor first before taking creatine.

How much should you take – and what about the 'loading phase'?

Dr Richard Kreider Phd gave a formula for working out how much creatine to take at first and then for daily maintenance. Dr Kreider is professor and head of the Department of Health and Kinesiology at Texas A&M University. He has published more than 300 sports nutrition articles and abstracts in scientific journals.

He advises that we initially increase muscle creatine stores by taking 0.3g per kg of bodyweight per day. Take this amount for 5-7 days and then simply take 3g-5g per day to maintain creatine stores. So an 80kg guy would take 24-25g for the first week and then reduce it to 5g daily. Or a 65kg woman would take 20g for the first week and then cut down to between 3g and 5g per day.

Stir Up Your Training Performance With Coffee

A cuppa coffee – without the sugar and cream – is an excellent pre-workout drink. It is a much healthier, safer choice than energy drinks.

A simple black coffee an hour before your workout can provide the following benefits:

- **Increased energy** – the high caffeine levels in coffee can provide a perfect power-up shortly before you hit the gym.

- **More fat loss** – coffee, when consumed before a workout, can cause fatty acids to be used for energy rather than glycogen. The caffeine content also speeds up metabolism, which means more fat is burned throughout the day.

- **Better performance** – coffee can be the difference between squeezing out a few more reps in the gym, or shaving a few seconds off your running time.

This was proven back in 1992 when a group of athletes were given 3g of coffee before a 1500m treadmill run. The study, published in the British Journal of Sports Medicine, showed that those who drank the coffee finished their run 4.2 secs faster on average than the control group. Other research also points to coffee helping to improve focus, decrease muscle pain during your workouts and even having a positive effect on your memory. So, while coffee is often seen as a vice by some people, it can actually have a positive impact when it comes to your training. Black and organic is best, and it's best sticking with the following advice:

Don't go overboard. Health experts recommend that no more than 400mg of caffeine (roughly three mugs of coffee) is consumed per day, while the limit is half that amount for pregnant women. Side effects of excessive caffeine intake include an increased heart rate and insomnia. Coffee is also acidic and too much acidity in the body leads to inflammation. Chronic inflammation depresses the immune system and can lead to health problems. Stay balanced by including plenty of vegetables and fruits, and natural, whole foods.

Choose freshly-made coffee – made with organic coffee beans if possible. Quality coffee beans contain various nutrients and flavonoid antioxidants, which help maintain good health. The processing of roasted coffee granules robs coffee of these nutrients.

Cut out the sugar and cream - unless your coffee is black you're defeating the purpose. Sugar will not only spike your insulin levels – and come crashing down later – but too much of the white stuff is also converted into fatty acids in the liver. Meaning more fat on your belly, legs, arms...or wherever else you don't want it.

CHECKLIST

- A great pre-workout combo is black coffee and creatine.

- The coffee will help boost energy and burn fat, and can have a positive impact on your performance in the gym.

- Creatine can help you gain muscle mass by enhancing your performance, strength, and your recovery after training. It can also give your muscles a fuller look by drawing more water into the muscles.

- Begin a creatine 'loading phase' of taking around 0.3g per kg of bodyweight for 5-7 days.

- Creatine supplementation thereafter should be reduced to 3g-5g per day.

- I take creatine in cycles, two months on and one month off. People with gout are advised not to take creatine as it will worsen the condition. If you have any health issues consult your doctor first.

- A coffee (no sugar or cream) an hour before your workout can increase energy levels, boost performance and burn fat more efficiently.

- Due to its high caffeine content, you should drink no more than 3 mugs of coffee per day. Choose freshly ground organic brand of coffee rather than instant, which has been stripped of its antioxidants and isn't as effective.

Chapter 11:

Post-workout Nutrition

When I first started out lifting weights when I was aged 16 I didn't have a clue about what I should be eating to try and build muscle. I can remember my friend Bryan and I training with a weight bench in his gran's house. Within seconds of finishing our last rep we were drinking pints of milk and wolfing down slice after slice of wafer thin honey roast ham. Wasn't exactly the tastiest combo but I'd read somewhere that milk helps you build muscle. These days I don't drink the stuff at all, but it's important to underline that it's not just what you eat, but when too.

The **two hour period** following your workout is prime time for making the most of your gym efforts. Ori Hofmekler, world leading sports nutritionist and author, describes it as the 'window of opportunity' for maximising muscle growth. Your body will temporarily be in a catabolic (muscle wasting) state following each weight training session. This is because the strain of intense exercise triggers the release of stress hormone cortisol in the body, which breaks down muscle tissue.

Doesn't sound good, right? But this biological process actually sets you up for flipping it into an anabolic (muscle building) state through proper nutrition afterwards. By flooding your body with the right nutrients – within the right timeframe – you halt the catabolic process and kickstart some serious muscle building as your body begins the growth and recovery phase following tough work done in the gym.

Feed Your Hungry Muscles Twice Within The Window Of Opportunity

The sooner we switch from catabolic to anabolic the better for muscle growth. This is where two post-workout 'feeds' come into play.

'Feed' 1

Within 30 mins of your workout: feed your muscles with fast assimilating protein to start the muscle building process. I recommend a plant-based protein shake, such as brown rice or vegan blend protein powder. Mixed with water, these are really easy for the body to absorb without any digestive issues.

'Feed' 2

60-90 minutes later: eat a healthy meal with a good balance of protein, complex carbs and healthy fats. These should come from the food sources mentioned in chapter 4. Not a good cook? There are tons of excellent cook books out there.

My book *'Meal Prep: 50 Simple Recipes For Health & Fitness Nuts'* has plenty of recipes that are ready in less than 30 minutes - and it also provides a breakdown of calories, protein, carbs and fats for each meal.

CHECKLIST

- The <u>two hour period</u> following your workout is prime time for making the most of your gym efforts.

- Aim for two 'feeds' (which is really just a shake and one meal) in this 'window of opportunity' for maximising muscle growth.

- I recommend a plant-based protein powder shake with water 30 minutes after finishing your workout.

- Then 60-90 minutes after your shake have a nutritious meal composed of good sources of protein, complex carbs and healthy fats as described in chapter 4.

Chapter 12:

Supplements: The Good, The Bad & The Useless

There's bodybuilding. And there's building a strong, healthy body. I class the two completely differently. I'd never consider myself a bodybuilder. A meathead bodybuilder probably wouldn't consider me a bodybuilder either. I'm cool with that. I'm just a guy who lifts heavy weights - and my health is of the utmost importance.

In my experience, I've seen too many bodybuilders put aesthetics, competition and their egos before their health. Just to get ahead, to try and be bigger or better than others, while not really thinking about any long-term consequences. Firstly, anyone who even considers taking steroids for a better body is not only a meathead, but a plain moron. You become fake, a fraud...and I won't bore you with the ball-shrinkingly frightening health dangers.

Secondly, anyone who takes other unnatural, synthetic pills, powders or liquids without properly doing their homework should also receive a 'moron' tattoo along with their gym membership.

"Take care of your body, it's the only place you have to live." – Jim Rohn.

Truth is: you don't need to waste your money on a bunch of supplements, dodgy or otherwise, to achieve the great body you want. A clean, healthy whole foods diet can provide virtually all you need. Having said that, there are still a handful of natural supplements that'll help you get the job done much more efficiently and effectively. I'll detail the 'essentials' and 'extras' I use to supplement my weight training program - and properly look after my body. They're safe, natural and opting for these will not only bring you excellent results, but it'll save you time, experimenting with garbage products, and a heck of a lot of money.

In part two of this chapter we'll also cover pre-workout and post-workout nutrition, which can be a headache for even the most experienced weightlifter. I'll share my 'ultimate pre-workout combo' for peak performance in the gym, aswell as tips on what to consume afterwards to gain the most from your monster gym efforts.

'The Essentials' – stock up on these whenever you get the chance

Multi-vitamin and mineral tablet

The body uses vitamins and minerals to repair and replace cells. We simply cannot function without these nutrients. The standard Western diet and the processing of food strips what we eat of its goodness. The result? Vitamin and mineral deficiencies. These deficiencies lead to various health problems. For example, if you lack vitamin B12 you'll likely feel tired, out of breath, or develop headaches.

It's like a car that needs oil and the warning light comes on. The body gives us plenty of warning signs too and it's up to us to give the body what it needs before it breaks down. But even eating plenty of organic fruit and veg isn't necessarily enough to cover all vitamin and mineral bases. So buying a good multivitamin and mineral supplement is a wise investment for foundational health.

Creatine

This could well be your weightlifting best friend. As described earlier, creatine has been proven to be effective in improving performance in weightlifters and other athletes. It increases the body's ability to produce energy more rapidly, meaning you can train harder – and for longer. Did I mention the benefits of fuller muscles, or enhanced recovery after workouts too? Creatine is an amino acid that's found in various foods and is naturally produced by the body too.

Plant-based protein powder

No I'm NOT talking about whey isolate protein powder. I ain't a fan of the usual type of protein that 98% of weightlifters/athletes/gym-goers drink to help build muscle. In my experience, some (not all) brands of whey protein are highly processed, contain chemicals and additives, and are acidic which makes it harder to digest and it has been argued that they can damage your health in the long term.

Myself and several friends suffered digestive problems after years of guzzling whey protein shakes. When we switched to an organic plant-based protein powder all the issues stopped. Plant-based protein powders are much more alkaline and easily absorbed by the body. My advice is to ditch whey protein, buy the plant-based stuff instead. You'll likely save yourself, your toilet and anyone within a 1 metre radius of you the pain of your constipation, diarrhoea and toxic farts.

Magnesium oil

Magnesium plays so many roles in the healthy functioning of our bodies, and is crucial for sports performance and recovery. But this mineral is also very easily depleted in our fast-paced, stressful lives. Intense exercise, such as heavy weight training can also further lower levels of magnesium and therefore it's a very wise move to supplement with magnesium oil. Dr Mark Sircus, author of Transdermal Magnesium Therapy, refers to magnesium as "by far the most important mineral in the body".

When it comes to performance: the body's main energy source ATP (adenosine triphosphate) must be bound to a magnesium ion in order to be biologically active. A deficiency in magnesium can therefore impair athletic performance. When it comes to recovery: supplementing with magnesium oil is hugely beneficial for people lifting weights because it relaxes and soothes sore muscles, speeding up recovery times after tough workouts.

It's also an amazing aid for a deep, restful sleep as it calms the nervous system by inhibiting the major stress hormones cortisol and adrenaline. Proper sleep is extremely important for muscle development and overall health. Spraying magnesium chloride oil on to the skin has been shown to be most effective for absorption.

'The Extras' – beneficial but not necessary if you don't have the cash

ZMA (Zinc, Magnesium, Vitamin B6)

This combination of two minerals and one vitamin is a potent mix for recovery and growth because it assists in achieving deep levels of sleep and hormone production. Training hard in the gym consistently can lower levels of testosterone, as can the stresses of everyday life.

ZMA has been clinically proven to increase anabolic hormone levels and muscle strength in athletes. Studies have shown that it can increase the testosterone levels of men by around one third.

Greens powder

We all know how good vegetables are for us. But let's be honest, most of us don't eat anywhere near enough of them. Even those who do eat plenty are probably not getting enough nutrients from them because over-cooking strips vegetables of vitamins, minerals and natural enzymes.

This is where a greens powder supplement can make all the difference. Packed with antioxidants and phytonutrients, this supplement is powerful for cleansing the entire body and protecting your cells. This can boost your immune system, improve digestion, and support overall health and wellbeing.

Digestive enzymes

Enzymes are produced by the body to break down our food properly and absorb the nutrients. They're also found in whole unprocessed foods such as fruit and veg. There are two problems: first, the body can struggle when faced with a constant influx of processed junk food and large volumes of animal protein, as found in the typical Western diet.

Heartburn, bloating, too much gas etc are all signs the body is having a hard time digesting what's been eaten. Secondly, cooking also robs foods of their natural enzymes. Digestive enzyme supplements can assist the body in breaking down larger volumes of food, such as cooked main meals. This means you get more out of what you eat, which of course provides the nutrients needed for muscle growth - and optimal health.

CHECKLIST

- The 'essentials' supplements are: multivitamin and mineral tablets, creatine, plant-based protein powder and magnesium oil.

- Multivitamins and minerals: these are important for addressing nutritional deficiencies that are common in the typical western diet and building good foundational health.

- Protein powder: choose an organic plant-based option, such as brown rice or vegan blend, over whey isolate protein. Not only because it is a highly absorbable form of protein, but because it's alkaline and therefore kinder to your insides than other highly processed, acidic brands.

- Magnesium oil: the huge role magnesium plays in sports performance, recovery and overall health is not widely known. It's also very easily depleted, especially following intense training. Stay one step ahead and look after your body well by supplementing with this magic mineral.

- The 'extras' supplements – if you've got the cash – are: ZMA capsules, greens powder and digestive enzymes.

Conclusion

I don't think anything I've explained in this book is hard to understand or follow. That's exactly the point. Proper nutrition/a clean diet/a healthy way of eating...whatever you want to call it...should be straightforward and easy to maintain. I take the same approach with my strength training programs too.

Otherwise, we end up in a never ending cycle of becoming temporarily enslaved to a fad diet >> making progress >> inevitably having a major blowout >> losing our way and feeling like crap >> beating ourselves up >> and then it's back to square one.

Does it not make more sense to just get all the basics right consistently? You know, like...

- Cutting down on sugar

- Limiting the booze

- Eating more vegetables and fruit

- Keeping an eye on your calories

- Drinking plenty of water and taking a vitamin and mineral supplement every day

Doing all of the above isn't hard work. Making good food choices – as described in chapter 4 – Monday-Friday ain't that difficult either. Especially when you can relax a bit and enjoy treats at the weekend. None of that sounds like a diet to me. It's simply a healthy eating lifestyle and will provide your body with what it needs as you progress on your strength training program.

As for training itself, I've experimented with all sorts of foods, drinks and supplements to give me fuel and boost my performance in the gym. Forget all these dodgy energy drinks or hyped-up supplements, a black coffee and creatine is the way forward. My energy and strength levels go through the roof with this combo.

If you're overweight then I'd go only with the coffee and leave out the creatine until you're close to your target weight. This is because creatine pulls water into your muscles and water retention isn't what you want.

As for the coffee, make sure it's black and go for a freshly made organic brew instead of instant. Remember to fully capitalise on your gym efforts by having two post-workout feeds within the two hour 'window of opportunity'. I have my plant-based protein powder shake 30 minutes after finishing my workout, and then follow this up around 60 minutes later with a nutritious meal such as oatcakes and tuna mayonnaise, or one of my special calorific super shakes!

You don't necessarily need to blow your cash on supplements to help you build muscle, strip fat and get in better overall shape. But, as I mentioned in the last chapter, there are some essentials and non-essentials which I use to complement my training regime and optimise my health. They're all completely natural, fairly cheap, and are worth every penny.

I hope you've enjoyed reading this book and it helps you become a stronger, better, healthier version of yourself. If you have any questions about anything in the book feel free to email me at: marc@weighttrainingistheway.com

Also, I'd be massively, ridiculously, eternally grateful if you left me a review of this book on Amazon.

Right, enough reading. Get back to the gym!

All the best, Marc McLean.

About The Author

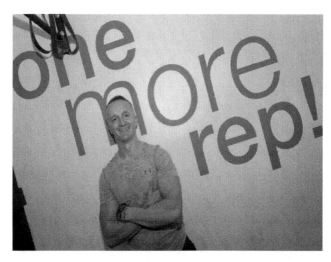

Marc McLean is a 35-year-old author and online personal training and nutrition coach from Loch Lomond in Scotland. He owns Weight Training Is The Way and is a health and fitness writer for leading websites including The Good Men Project, Mind Body Green, and Healthgreatness.com

Marc loves...climbing Munros (aka the biggest hills) in Scotland, peanut butter, amazing scenery, the Rocky movies, lifting heavy things, blueberries, Daft Punk, tennis, travelling and having a laugh with his mates.

Marc hates...bad manners, funerals, cardio, and all drivers who don't indicate.

You can connect with Marc here:

Email: marc@weighttrainingistheway.com

Website: www.weighttrainingistheway.com

Facebook: www.facebook.com/weighttrainingistheway

Instagram: www.instagram.com/weight_training_is_the_way

Strength Training 101 Book Series

This book is the second in the 'Strength Training 101' series by Marc McLean. The others include:

Book 1: *Strength Training NOT Bodybuilding: How To Build Muscle & Burn Fat…Without Morphing Into A Bodybuilder*

Book 3: *Meal Prep: 50 Simple Recipes For Health & Fitness Nuts.*

Book 4: *Burn Fat Fast: Ridiculously Effective Flab Busting Secrets Revealed.*

Book 5: *Strength Training For Women: Burn Fat Effectively…And Sculpt The Body You've Always Dreamed Of.*

Bibliography / Further Reading / References

Essentials of Strength Training and Conditioning, 3rd edition – Baechle, Earle.

The Warrior Diet – Ori Hofmekler.

Eat Stop Eat – Brad Pilon.

The Power Of Habit - Charles Duhigg.

Paul M La Bounty, Bill I Campbell, Jacob Wilson, Elfego Galvan, John Berardi,

Susan M Kleiner, Richard B Kreider,
Jeffrey R Stout,Tim Ziegenfuss, Marie Spano, Abbie Smith and Jose Antonio. March 2011. International Society of Sports Nutrition position stand: meal frequency.
http://www.jissn.com/content/8/1/4

MM Manore. August 2005. Exercise and the Institute of Medicine recommendations for nutrition.
http://www.ncbi.nlm.nih.gov/pubmed/16004827

R Estruch, E Ros, J Salas-Salvado, M Isabel-Covas, D Pharm, D Corella, F Aros, E Gomez-Gracia, V Ruiz-Gutierrez, M Fiol, J Lapetra, RM Lamuela-Raventos, L Serra Majem, X Pinto, J Pasora, M A Munoz, J V Sorli, J A Martinez, M A Martinez-Gonzalez. Primary Prevention of Cardiovascular Disease with a Mediterranean Diet. April 2013.
http://www.nejm.org/doi/full/10.1056/NEJMoa1200303

P J Atherton, T Etheridge, P W Watt, D Wilkinson, A Selby, D Rankin, K Smith, M J Rennie. November 2010. Muscle full effect after oral protein: time-dependent concordance and discordance between human muscle protein synthesis and mTORC1 signaling.
http://www.ncbi.nlm.nih.gov/pubmed/20844073

J D Wiles, S R Bird, J Hopkins and M Riley. June 1992. Effect of caffeinated coffee on running speed, respiratory factors, blood lactate and perceived exertion during 1500-m treadmill running. British Journal of Sports Medicine. https://www.ncbi.nlm.nih.gov/pmc/articles/PMC1478936/

C Rae, A L Digney, S R McEwan, T C Bates. October 2003. Oral creatine monohydrate supplementation improves brain performance: a double-blind, placebo-controlled, cross-over trial. https://www.ncbi.nlm.nih.gov/pubmed/14561278

R V Santos, R A Bassit, E C Caperuto, L F Costa Rosa. September 2004. The effect of creatine supplementation upon inflammatory and muscle soreness markers after a 30km race.

https://www.ncbi.nlm.nih.gov/pubmed/15306159

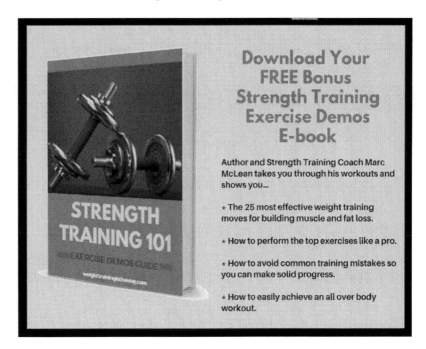

Visit The Website Below To Access Your Copy

www.weighttrainingistheway.com

36571375R10051

Made in the USA
Middletown, DE
15 February 2019